W9-AUA-242

GIANT STEPS

GIANT STEPS

The Story of One Boy's Struggle to Walk

GILBERT M. GAUL

St. Martin's Press   New York

GIANT STEPS: THE STORY OF ONE BOY'S STRUGGLE TO WALK. Copyright © 1993 by Gilbert M. Gaul. All rights reserved. Printed in the United States of America. No part of this book may be used or reproduced in any manner whatsoever without written permission except in the case of brief quotations embodied in critical articles or reviews. For information, address St. Martin's Press, 175 Fifth Avenue, New York, N.Y. 10010.

Design by Judith A. Stagnitto

Library of Congress Cataloging-in-Publication Data

Gaul, Gilbert M.
    Giant steps / Gilbert M. Gaul.
      p. cm.
    "A Thomas Dunne book."
    ISBN 0-312-08729-2
    1. Gaul, Cary. 2. Spina bifida—Patients—Biography. I. Title.
RJ496.S74G384   1993
362.1'97375—dc20
[B]   92-33827
                                        CIP

First Edition: January 1993
10 9 8 7 6 5 4 3 2 1

For Cary,
whose sweet, stubborn strength has always inspired me,
and all of the other brave children of the world.

And Cathy and Greg,
who have shared this journey and have made this
family whole.

Contents

GIANT STEPS

ONE

A Journey of Days

I think of you all the time. In the _morning, you are there beside me when I crawl out of bed. During the day, you suddenly appear around the corner, freezing my thoughts. At night, you hover above me in my dreams, a tiny, whirling presence in the shadows, calling me, drawing me near. When I wake, I pull you close so you are safe. I taste your skin, so sweet and sour and new, smell the familiar clean powder on your clothes, swim in the nonsense gurgles of your conversations, catch the happy bubbles you blow, one after another, then watch helplessly as you slip away from me, my voice rolling back and away from you, as you soar._

—JOURNAL ENTRY
SEPTEMBER 1986

In the waking hours of a damp April morning six years ago, my wife Cathy and I gathered up our sleeping five-year-old son, Gregory, depositing him in his pajamas at a friend's house, and headed off to a hospital nearly ten miles away to deliver our second baby.

Once there, things began to unravel very quickly. Our unborn son, who had been largely quiet his first nine months, chose these fading moments to turn tail-down. This, in turn, prompted Ronald Jaffe, who was on weekend call for Cathy's regular obstetrician, to strongly recommend a caesarean section. "In a situation like this, at the last minute, you want to avoid any undue risk of damage," he explained. "It's really the only way to go."

We quickly agreed—the memory of a friend's breached and broken baby all too fresh in our minds—and Cathy was wheeled off to a nearby surgical suite. I remained behind in what was to have been our birthing room, a cheerful little spot with flowered wallpaper, rocking chair, and lace curtains, and waited until a nurse came for me. Everything was going to be just fine, I reassured myself. Caesarean's are no big deal. Doctors perform thousands of them daily, often under far more difficult conditions. A few snips, a tug, and out pops the baby. Still, some part of me feared the unknown, and I offered up a prayer, asking God to protect my wife and unborn child.

Cathy was already draped, prepped, and numbed from the waist down by the time I was led into the compact, mint-green room with a single operating table at the end of the hall. There, a solicitous nurse with a firm grip directed me alongside my wife and then quickly retreated to the other side of the room, where Jaffe and an assistant busied themselves checking their instruments, and an anesthesiologist, masked and focused, fiddled with a series of stainless-steel knobs behind Cathy's head. I reached for Cathy's hand and gave it a squeeze, and she squeezed back. The good soldier, she was smiling nervously. But I knew better. She hated needles and was terrified by the thought of someone slicing her. Here, in what must be her worst nightmare come true, she was subject to both.

I was curious about the surgery and watched intently as Jaffe made a horizontal incision across Cathy's swollen abdomen and neatly worked his way through muscle and fat to her uterus. "If you have a camera, now's the time to get it ready," his assistant advised me. "I'll give you the signal."

Moments later, as I positioned myself, Jaffe suddenly glanced over at me and shook his head. The tense, birdlike gesture filled me with terror. My first thought was that the baby was dead. Yet how could this be? Less than an hour before, we had listened to its miraculous heartbeat fill the room with a deep, sweet song. I reassured myself our baby couldn't slip that quickly from our grasp, could not fly away from us without a sign.

"What is it?" Cathy's voice suddenly rushed up at us. Low on the operating table, she could not see our faces above the drape, but she could read the silence that had replaced our idle chatter. "Something's wrong, isn't it? Something is wrong with our baby."

I looked to Jaffe for help. Once more, he shook his head. There was an unmistakable warning in his dark, fatigued eyes. Instinctively, I reached for Cathy's hand again and grabbed hold. I sensed the warm blood draining quickly from my face, rushing away like a forgotten underground stream, and suddenly felt cold.

"There appears to be a cele on the baby's lower back," Jaffe said in a low and measured voice, which left no mistaking the gravity of the situation, "and there's a problem with his feet."

With that vague yet chilling announcement, our new son, whom we had decided to name Cary, was swept from Cathy's womb, his umbilical cord snipped, and then he was quickly wrapped in a green hospital linen. It all happened so quickly, Cathy didn't see a thing, which I am sure is what Jaffe intended, and for which I am now thankful. The accidental glimpse I was afforded, however brief, exploded like a hot beam of light in my face, blinding me then, now, and quite probably forever with an image of a splintered, twisted baby. A wet, purplish sac, the size of an adult fist, clung to Cary's lower back like a barnacle. Jaffe had called this a cele, which was meaningless to me at the time. Still, I did not have to be a doctor to know it was something to be feared. Something raw and dangerous. So, too, Cary's legs, which dangled listlessly from the rest of his trunk, like tiny sticks. And his cartilaginous feet, which darted inward at horrific right angles. Deep in my soul I felt a hole opening and a firestorm rush through.

Cary was secreted across the hallway in a Level Two neonatal intensive-care nursery, one of only three such specialty facilities in southern New Jersey. There, he was bundled in a fresh set of linens, given a snug white cap that reminded me of a tiny longshoreman's, and placed carefully on his side in a temperature-controlled incubator, called an isolette. A small scrum of nurses and residents hovered over him, performing tests and talking in hushed tones. Machines, flashing lights, and electronic impulses recorded each thrust and flutter, kicking out a dizzying history of patchwork lines and jagged peaks. Ordinarily, in my job as a medical economics writer, I might have been impressed by this awesome concentration of expensive technology. But now I felt confused and ragged, as though I had been drugged and set free in some sort of high-tech dog kennel.

Every so often, one of the nurses would break free from the commotion to reassure me that Cary was comfortable and in no immediate danger. What did that mean: no immediate danger? That Cary would survive the morning, the day, the night? What about the gelatinous mass on his back and his twisted feet—were these also minor problems in the exaggerated calculus of trauma? Didn't they understand the raw urgency of the moment? The message of all these exotic machines? The fire in my gut?

When an opportunity presented itself, I elbowed my way forward for a better look. He was bundled so tightly, all I could see was Cary's face. Ah, but what a face it was, full and pink, with striking blue eyes that locked on me and wouldn't let go, lips pursed as if in a kiss, and a button nose, a clear gift from his mother, handed down through generations, a brilliant signature stroke now sweetly accepted.

I took these fleeting but joyous images and shared them greedily as I hurried back and forth between the busy nursery and my trembling, isolated wife. I did my best to reassure and comfort Cathy. Yet I knew there was no way to beat back the suffocating pain and shock she now felt.

Twice while Cathy was being stitched back up, I'd had to retreat to the hallway to catch my breath. Alone, I shrank against the cold tile and sorted through the images spinning inside my head. But the more I searched for answers, the more I became tangled in my own chaotic thoughts, the more the world twisted wildly around me, looping forward one moment, then suddenly jerking backward, obscenely cruel and disconnected. Each time, I was pulled back to reality by the sound of Jaffe's voice politely asking a nurse to please go check on the father. I told myself that I couldn't allow them to find me collapsed this way. I had to be strong for Cathy and the child. They were depending on me to gather information and make decisions. I could not and would not let them down. Even if, inwardly, I was whirling like an out-of-control top. Even if all I wanted to do was shrink away, to cry out like a wounded animal and nurse my blinding fear.

A little later, I accompanied Cathy when she was wheeled into a nearby recovery room. She was shaking from the aftereffects of the epidural block she had been given and was dazed and weepy. Jaffe came by and reassured her that Cary was in good hands and in no pain. One of our pediatricians would arrive shortly, and then a decision would be made about what to do next. Cary's problems were serious enough that they could not be treated here. He would have to be transported to one of the children's hospitals in nearby Philadelphia, where he would probably undergo surgery to repair the lesion on his back. It was impossible to predict anything after that, Jaffe said. The specialists there would be able to give us more information.

Nurses followed Jaffe with blankets and kind words. We clung to their boundless hope, reassured by their experience, and their unanimous view that Cary was an alert, vital baby. I helped to wrap Cathy in the blankets and held her close. But still she could not stop shaking. "I feel so cold," she repeated numbly. I pulled her closer, afraid, helpless, and together we sobbed quietly. It seemed we remained that way, locked in our shared grief, a long time, although I know that was impossible because it was only a few ticks, a blink, and a whisper, before I heard my name called and I felt my heart begin to crack again.

Moments later, I found myself back in the hallway, face to face with Ofelia Mangubat, a member of our pediatricians' group. Small and painfully shy at times, I liked Mangubat and found her to have a good, kind heart, no small saving grace in any doctor. But now her face was gray with worry as we exchanged tired hellos and she took up the unwelcome task of explaining what had gone wrong.

Our baby had been born with a serious birth defect known as myelomeningocele, she said, a condition in which the embryonic neural tube does not close completely and many of the nerves below that point are damaged or missing. Cary would be paralyzed and would suffer other problems, but only specialists would be able to say how severe they would be. So she had arranged for him to be taken by ambulance across the Delaware River to Children's Hospital in Philadelphia as soon as possible. There, he would undergo many tests and be operated on as well, perhaps even today, she said.

Mangubat's words raced in circles around my brain. How could this be? Why us? We were a healthy, conscientious couple. We didn't smoke or drink. We had never done drugs or engaged in any of the other high-risk behaviors one typically associates with the parents of low-birthweight infants and children with birth defects. And yet . . . and yet, unless I was dreaming, it apparently was all too real. "Will he ever be able to walk?" I asked weakly.

Mangubat shook her head. "These children, because of their paralysis, do not walk," she said, quickly adding, "He also has severe clubfeet, which must be fixed."

Why bother if he can't walk? I wondered. But this was more spasm than question, a tick of memory, not reason, quickly buried by its own weight. Afraid, I asked anyway, "Will he be retarded?"

Mangubat blinked. "Yes, there's a good chance he may be retarded." She sighed. "There are numerous complications."

I thanked her and staggered back into the nursery. Cary had his eyes closed now and appeared to be sleeping. His tiny chest fluttered against the linen like a gentle wave. Watching him, I drifted between utter fear and an overwhelming desire to disappear. As Mangubat's brief descriptions echoed within me, a mental image rose up of a child strapped to a wheelchair, staring blankly out at the world, never able to run or laugh or even cut his own birthday cake. I shuddered at this thought and tried to push it out of my mind. I did not know if I was strong enough to shield and protect such a child. Or would the Sisyphean demands and disappointment swallow me whole? Try as I might, I could not will forth an answer. It was too soon. All I had were questions.

I was unsure how much of this information I should share with Cathy. In nine years of marriage, my wife had continually surprised me with her courage and resiliency, but now she was exhausted and shocked. Her puffy eyes read my anxiety. "He's going to live, isn't he?"

"Yes, he is." I tried to explain what Mangubat had told me in the hallway, blunting the more painful edges.

"Promise me," Cathy said, fumbling for my hands, "no matter what we have to do, or how much, we won't let this come between us?"

Tears had formed again at the corners of Cathy's eyes,

and I could feel her hands trembling. Mine, too. "I promise," I said, "nothing will ever come between us."

"Because if it does . . . I don't know what I would do."

"I won't let it. We can handle this. No matter what. I promise."

Years later, this vow would lodge in my throat each time I recalled Cary's birth. Because we had no answers, no idea what it would be like to raise a severely disabled child, we had clung to the only thing we had known, our deep and trusting love. That was understandable, if somewhat naive. We were flying blind during those first few hours and days, with no history or context, no way of realizing the demands and stress that the years ahead had in store for us. All we knew was what we could see: our paralyzed son and the clamorous rush of modern medicine around him. Emotionally, we drifted between feeling dazed and numb, as though we had fast-forwarded into a nightmare and were now stuck there.

Nor could we possibly know that these first few hours, fearsome as they were, would in some ways be among the easiest of our journey. Cary was damaged and needed surgery; at least that much was relatively clear-cut. Later on, few decisions would be so certain, few of the roads we traveled so straight and smooth.

Medicine, we would discover, is a far more imprecise science than generally imagined by outsiders, especially when it comes to treating children with physical defects. Dominated by big-ticket surgeons and ever more elaborate forms of technology, its focus is on curing, not caring for the chronic needs of children whose muscles aren't strong enough to support them, whose bladders don't drain properly, and whose brains don't "see" things right.

Such lesser chores are left to the acolytes—the nurses and therapists and school aides, who work for a fraction of physicians' salaries, yet often make the biggest difference in these children's lives. Even then, most of the daily responsibilities fall squarely on the shoulders of parents, and especially the mothers.

We are a couple of ordinary patience and emotional limits. Yet, time and again, we discovered inner resources we didn't know we had. Cathy and I have gained strength from these moments, as well as newfound respect for one another. But there have also been moments when the demands pushed us over the edge, when we realized our energies were not as boundless as we had imagined or hoped. More than once, we have crawled off to bed beaten and exhausted to escape in a book or sleep.

Fortunately, the next day has often brought relief, and along with it, some small gain or long-delayed milestone in Cary's development. We have treasured these days and have used them to replenish our empty stores. A sense of humor and perspective has also helped. Cathy is fond of saying, "Don't sweat the small stuff," which is not at all bad advice when dealing with the many and varied needs of a disabled child. Cary, whose stubborn personality is formidable and challenging, also appreciates a joke, and is known around our household as a wicked kidder. On more than one occasion, he has broken an otherwise tense situation by reducing us to belly laughs. These moments have helped us understand that, no matter how many challenges we face, we are a family first, with all of the joys and disappointments, victories and losses, bound together by a journey of days, each lived one at a time.

Of the one-million-plus American families in which a

chronically ill or disabled child resides, most will lead lives of quiet dignity this year. They will negotiate the highs and lows of their experience with everyday rectitude and an unflinching commitment to normalcy. Most will ask of society only that their children be given a fair chance, whether that means attending school, using community property, or just playing with the other kids in their neighborhoods. They will not expect to be singled out for special privileges, with a few small exceptions, such as being permitted parking closer to stores. Nor will the vast majority seek out the limelight or look to be anointed because of their differences. Most, frankly, will abhor such displays as patronizing and ultimately self-defeating.

A journey with any child is a series of bumps and tumbles and capers. The life of a disabled child is no different in this regard. Only the angles are sharper. The footings less sure. The milestones longer and pitched. The edges more subtle and dangerous. This is the story of one such child's journey. It is a journey marked by shock, hurt, hope, and joy, a story about family, medicine, and society. But most of all it is a story about watching a child work his way past numerous obstacles to master simple and large tasks as he engages the world around him and struggles to make it his.

Later that first morning, after the transport team arrived and had begun to ready Cary for his trip across the river to Children's Hospital, we were visited by Rhoda Burns, a second-year medical resident on duty with the team this dreary Sunday morning.

"Mr. and Mrs. Gaul," Burns said, inching her tall frame near us. "I was just with your son Cary. He's a beautiful baby."

"He is beautiful, isn't he?" Cathy said, grabbing hold of Rhoda Burns's words. "But I've barely seen him."

"We will bring him by before we leave."

"He's beautiful?"

"He is. He's a beautiful baby," Burns said.

Many doctors and nurses cared for us in the first few hours after Cary's birth, and all were generous and warm. Yet it was this relatively unpracticed newcomer who offered us the gift we needed when we were weakest. With her few simple words and unpretentious manner, Rhoda Burns gave us reason to hope.

TWO

The Kindness of Strangers

On the night of Cary's birth, I drove across the Walt Whitman Bridge to Philadelphia to visit our newborn son at Children's Hospital, a sprawling, well-heeled, layer cake of a hospital that also is one of America's finest pediatric speciality centers.

There, amid an incongruous clutter of broken toys and expensive medical equipment, I found Cary tucked away in a corner of the fifth floor in a six-crib cubbyhole known as the Infant Transitional Unit, or Infant Trans for short. As its name suggests, the Infant Transitional Unit serves as a kind of medical catchall, lodging babies who have been in intensive care but are well enough now to be cared for in a less-critical setting, or in cases such as Cary's, newborns who require close handling but aren't considered to be critically ill.

This particular night, Infant Trans was home to two infants with breathing disorders known as sleep apnea, a newborn boy with a blocked intestine, a baby girl with undiagnosed neurological damage, Cary, and two older boys who had been delivered several months premature by drug-addicted mothers. Now nearly toddlers, the boys had become wards of the hospital, or as they are known in medical circles, "boarder babies," at no small cost to society. During Cary's two weeks here, one boy's mother visited him for an hour, nearly all of which she spent sleeping or watching television. The other boy's mother had yet to appear, and the nurses said she was rumored to be living in a crack house. Social workers at the hospital were working desperately to place the boys in foster homes, but thus far hadn't been successful.

I located Cary in an isolette creased against a corner window looking out on West Philadelphia and the University of Pennsylvania's dusty red-brick buildings. His tiny body was crowded with wires and an odd assortment of other lines taped to his wrists and ankles. My heart sank; our little boy was literally wired for sound. An overhead monitor recorded each flutter and blip of his heart, setting off a nerve-shattering caterwaul whenever he stopped breathing even momentarily.

"Oh, these things will drive you nuts," Marion Logue, a bright, young, energetic nurse assigned to Cary casually remarked. Each time the alarm sounded, Logue or another nurse hustled over from the nurses' station, checked to see if he was breathing normally and then reset the alarm. "Sometimes it goes off if a baby just coughs or holds his breath and we end up running around all night. But then with the apnea babies there's always that chance," Logue said.

Several IV poles towered over Cary like high-tension lines. Through these clear plastic tubes, he received antibiotics to ward off a potentially lethal infection, glucose for nourishment, and liquids to prevent dehydration. The medical chart attached to the side of his steamy incubator reported that he had arrived at the unit shortly after noon and was the 8-lb., 5-oz. product of a full-term uncomplicated pregnancy to a thirty-two-year-old Gravida II, Para I mother. For insurance purposes, our son was identified as patient J264805.

The nurses had propped Cary on his side so an overhead tube could drip saline solution into the bandage covering his lesion. The thin, gelatinous membrane had to be moist, Logue explained, to prevent it from cracking and becoming infected before surgery. An infection at this juncture would spread rapidly up Cary's spinal cord to his brain and possibly kill him, she said.

Despite all of the hardware, the glare of the lights, the occasional blaring alarm, and the near-tropical temperature, Cary slept soundly. In time, I too, became accustomed to the busy surroundings. Pulling up a rocking chair next to the isolette, I poked my disinfected hands (signs everywhere reminded parents to wash before touching) through the small round portals and gently massaged my son's splintery legs. I was advised that Cary probably did not feel this. But the way he fixed his magnificent blue eyes on me suggested otherwise. Besides, it made *me* feel good.

During feedings, I was permitted to take Cary from his isolette and give him a bottle of his mother's thawed breast milk, which I transported daily between the hospitals and which he gulped down greedily. Later, after he was moved to a crib, I could retrieve him any time I liked. He seemed to especially enjoy being held late at night, when we would gently rock back and forth and watch the hospital wind down at the end of another busy day.

The first two weeks of Cary's life were probably the most difficult and exhausting of our lives. For Cathy, it meant being separated from her baby, for nearly a week, not knowing at any moment whether he was happy or sad, safe or facing some crisis; for me, it meant racing between hospitals, wrestling with medical decisions, and juggling child-care arrangements and family matters back at home.

Yet, strangely enough, these first weeks were also marked by interludes when I felt totally at peace with the world, moments when just holding my baby was enough and it was possible to forget all of the recent traumas and enjoy Cary the way a father would any newborn son.

The day after Cary was born I met with Edward Charney, a developmental pediatrician and the director of the center's program for children born with myelomeningocele, or as it is more popularly known, spina bifida.

Medium built, with a droopy, wraparound mustache and dark, wiry hair, Charney bore a slight resemblance to the actor Elliot Gould. He also leaned toward the movie star's quick, glib manner, which many but not all of the parents found a refreshing change to the intensely serious, button-down culture of academic medicine that dominated CHOP.

Charney had already been by to see Cary and had also spoken with several specialists who had visited our son earlier while on their rounds. As the overall case manager of Cary's medical care, it was now his job to pass along these findings.

"The good news," he said, fidgeting behind a cluttered desk, "is that Cary appears to be a strong, motivated little guy. He moves his hips voluntarily, which is a good sign, and appears to also have some control of his quadriceps and maybe his hamstrings. That's less certain because I wasn't really testing him." Charney eyed me to see if I was following thus far, and I nodded that I was. "He doesn't move his ankles, and there's a question of sensation in his lower extremities. He may have some feeling in his knees or his lower thighs. Again, I'm not sure. In terms of involvement, I would say he is approximately L-two or L-three."

"What does that mean?"

"Okay, good question. What that means is his lesion occurred either at the second or third vertebra of the lumbar section of his spine. That is where the neural tube interrupted and nerves below that point were affected. Actually, it's a pretty common area. He's what we might call a middle-of-the-roader."

I had brought along a spiral notebook and used it now to jot down what the doctor said. I imagined this would help me later when I tried to recall the conversation for Cathy. But playing reporter also helped to distract and blunt the full force of Charney's words. I heard him and understood what he was saying, yet a part of me was also detached, watching the proceedings from a safe distance. "What nerves will be affected?" I heard this other voice ask.

Charney leaned back in his chair. His eyes darted nervously as he measured me. "I can't say because it's too early," he said. "What I can tell you, and this is very general, is based on all of the other kids we have seen with levels of involvement similar to Cary's. But the caveat, again, is that it's not exact. No two kids are ever alike. They can have the same level of involvement but have totally different capabilities, different muscles, and make dramatically different progress. But within these parameters, I can give you a pretty good idea."

"All right."

"The two big things we focus on here are getting the kids up and walking and getting them out of diapers, so they can be socially accepted by their peers. As far as ambulating, Cary should be a walker when he gets older with the aid of braces and crutches. He will definitely need braces, at least initially probably up to his hips. The fact that he seems strong and determined should help. And in time we may be able to cut the bracing down. Again, I can't say how low or if it will even happen. It could be to mid-thigh, but I've also seen kids at his level of involvement go as low as their knees. We won't be able to know until we see how much control he has and that won't be for a year or two.

"As far as his bladder goes, there is almost a hundred percent probability he will have a problem because of the damage to his nerves," Charney said. "The goal will be to teach Cary what we call intermittent self-catheterization, which is where the children use a catheter to empty their bladder several times a day. About eighty percent of the kids are candidates for intermittent catheterization and are able to stay dry. I can't emphasize that enough because of the role it plays in socialization later on when these kids move into school. They already are ostracized because they look different, so it's terribly important, we've found, that they don't stand out in other ways. You definitely want to remove that social stigma."

To be sure, there would be other issues as we went along, Charney advised, but we would learn to deal with them one at a time. Because of his bladder problems, Cary would be prone to urinary-tract infections and would have to be monitored carefully, including undergoing periodic ultrasounds to make sure infections and a reflux of urine weren't damaging his kidneys, a potentially lethal problem among some young adults with spina bifida.

There was also a chance that Cary would be incontinent because of nerve damage. That could result in constipation, or worse, he might become impacted and require surgery. To avoid these pitfalls, his diet would have to be rich in fiber and fiber supplements. When he was older, say two or three, we could begin a bowel management program, using suppositories or enemas to empty his bowels on a regular schedule, usually once a day or every other day. In time, Cary might learn to recognize his body's signals and do away with these props. It was impossible to be more specific at this point and too soon to worry about, Charney emphasized. It also was probably the single most frustrating aspect of caring for these children.

An orthopedic surgeon would correct Cary's clubfeet sometime in the next few months by cutting tendons that allowed the feet to straighten. Without this operation, his rigidly curved feet would not support the weight of his frame, and he wouldn't be able to walk. Over the years, Cary might also be especially susceptible to fractures and bruises because of his undersized legs and weakened bones, contractures of joints, tendons, and muscles that stiffened and shortened from underuse, dislocated hips because of muscle imbalances, pressure sores where his braces rubbed against his skin, and scoliosis, or curvature of the spine, although this problem was more common among girls.

In addition, he might suffer scarring of tissue where the lesion formed on his spinal cord. This became a problem as the child grew and the scarred tissue adhered to the cord instead of stretching normally. Although still poorly understood, "Tethered Cord Syndrome" was increasingly being associated with the sudden onset of a host of problems, including deterioration in walking ability, posture, and bowel control, Charney said.

About half of the children also exhibited learning disabilities in school, especially in the area of visual-perceptual skills, such as cutting with scissors and holding a pencil. It was unclear why these problems occurred, Charney said. One school of thought held that children with spina bifida suffer a compression of the hindbrain and brainstem, which stretches and distorts the pathways of certain nerves, garbling the incoming and outgoing signals. Other theorists believed the problems were the result of a general lag in development; when other children were walking and engaging the world eye-to-eye, toddlers with spina bifida were still crawling and overly dependent on their parents. The bottom line was no one knew. And because a child's brain isn't like a television, you couldn't just pop the back and wiggle a few wires until the picture improved. You had to sit and wait patiently and hope that the signal returned on its own.

As for Cary's overall intelligence, statistics showed that the majority of children born with spina bifida were not retarded, Charney explained. "They appear to have a reasonable distribution of intelligence, with most falling in the average range." Based on his examination earlier, Charney continued, Cary didn't appear to have suffered any obvious damage to his brain. He seemed bright and alert and very active, all of which were good signs.

I breathed a sigh of relief, recalling what Mangubat had told me less than twenty-four hours earlier. Why had she said those things? Most likely, she hadn't known better, hadn't ever seen a newborn with spina bifida, and had recalled a few odds and ends she had gleaned from medical texts or heard along the way. If Cary could think for himself and had normal intelligence, he could overcome a lot of other obstacles, I reasoned. He could go to school and get a job and live independently. His life might not be perfect, but it could be rewarding and have purpose. I locked onto this idea even as Charney was moving on to other, more immediate problems.

"At the moment," he said, "there are two issues that you and your wife have to decide—whether to surgically close the lesion on Cary's back and, should it be required, whether to insert a shunt to control hydrocephalus, or a buildup of fluid on the brain."

"What will happen if the lesion isn't closed?"

"Cary will almost certainly develop an infection. It could be sooner than later. Statistically, there would be an eighty percent chance of his dying."

"How soon would you want to do the operation?"

Charney smiled. "I wouldn't do it. If you agree, a neurosurgeon will operate within a day or two. We wouldn't want to wait any longer because of the risk.

"This is not a clear-cut decision," he continued. "You could decide to do nothing, in which case, Cary would probably die, almost certainly within the first year. Or you could go ahead. You are in a position that is not unlike—I don't know if you are familiar with it?—the Baby Jane Doe case, which got so much publicity several years ago."

In fact, I was familiar with the case through my job at *The Philadelphia Inquirer*, where I report on medical economics and health policy. It had involved a painful ethical and legal battle between government and Right-to-Life attorneys and the parents of a Long Island girl born with spina bifida and a series of other birth defects. Doctors had predicted that, even with surgery to close her lesion, the infant girl would be severely retarded and suffer numerous medical problems. The girl's parents had decided against the operation. Attorneys for the federal government had intervened in the case, questioning the parents' legal right to deny the surgery. Two years later, the Supreme Court had struck down the regulations the government had cited as its basis for intervening.

"All I am saying," Charney continued, as though reading my confusion, "is that if you and your wife decide to do nothing, I can't guarantee you that some external pressure will not be brought from outside the hospital. I'm not saying it will happen, but it could. I feel I would be remiss if I didn't tell you."

Charney's words startled me. Intellectually, I was appalled that outsiders could force their will on such a personal and painful decision. Yet the idea of allowing Cary to die had never crossed my mind. Perhaps if I had never seen his soft red mouth or held his tiny hands in mine I might have felt differently. But I had swum in our little boy's deep blue eyes; I had listened to his sweet heart-song and fed him his mother's milk. There was no way I could turn my back on him. Cary was a part of our family now, our history and blood. We would do anything to make him comfortable. And that included surgery to close his lesion.

Charney waved me off before I could answer. "Talk it

over with your wife. If she has any questions, or just wants to talk to me, she can call me from the hospital this evening." He wrote down his home number and gave it to me. "I would be happy to talk to her."

Charney had arranged for me to meet with Leslie Sutton, one of the hospital's neurosurgeons, who would explain the procedure to repair Cary's lesion. Before I left, however, he added one final thought:

"I know you're probably feeling a little overwhelmed right now. You wouldn't be normal if you weren't. Over time, what I've learned is that the emotions we see in clinic tend to be a reflection of the family unit and how it's doing. The families that had problems before seem to continue to have problems after having a baby with spina bifida. The stress of taking care of the child just brings the problems out in a more dramatic manner. Conversely, the families that were strong before seem to fare better overall. They support one another and balance the needs of the child against the needs of the family, and are able to maintain a sense of order in their lives. I'm not saying there aren't stresses; there are. Lots of them. But there's also a lot of good, too. Although, again, it's probably kind of tough to see that right now."

Charney's words, delivered with a familiar insider's pitch, cascaded through my brain as I made my way down a busy back stairwell frequented by the nurses and residents to Sutton's third-floor office.

Our family was strong and intact, I reassured myself. Not perfect or even near perfect. But caring and devoted and whole. Cathy and I had known one another for seventeen years, and had been married for nearly ten. We had overcome our share of obstacles and disappointments along the way and were still very much in love. The birth of our other son Gregory five years earlier had brought new excitement and challenges to our marriage. We had had to learn to balance our needs against the demands of a very bright and willful child. There had been the usual number of bumps and false starts. But in time we had eased into our roles as parents and had settled into a rewarding and happy life.

Cary's needs would be extraordinary by comparison. The operations, trips to doctors, and therapy sessions seemed daunting at this moment. Yet he was only an infant, barely twenty-four hours old. We would have time to get used to him, I reminded myself, and he to us. And as with any newborn, we would learn routines and shortcuts, become practiced at the more difficult tasks and share the caregiving. It wouldn't be easy. But it wouldn't be all work either. In return for all our work, we would gain a new member of our family and get to share in all of Cary's discoveries and milestones. For each setback, there was bound to be a reward, however small, a laugh or a word or some private moment of accomplishment to sustain us. Disciplined, at times even stoic, I was a firm believer that life was made up of these small moments of mastery and insight and joy, not blinding epiphanies and storybook endings. It was the nuances of character and delight in everyday experiences that carried our spirits and propelled us onward to greater things. This was my anthem. One day I hoped it might also be my son's.

THREE

Seeds

We are often told that first impressions are the most accurate. When in doubt, stick with one's initial reaction. Experience shows it will usually hold up. Leslie Sutton, I discovered, is an important exception to this rule.

My first meeting with the lanky neurosurgeon left me cold. Oh, there was no doubting Sutton's competence. It resonated in each carefully crafted sentence he spoke. Here was a superior talent. A worthy craftsman and an inquisitive mind. Vigilant but not reckless. In short, someone I could entrust Cary to without great fear.

The trouble was the good doctor's demeanor. Sutton was so practiced at the professional art of detachment, he might as well have been presenting a scientific paper to his colleagues. I found myself resenting his safe distance. Didn't he understand how I *felt*? The fine line I was treading between exhaustion and collapse? Couldn't he see I needed more than his crisp scientific bullets? Apparently not. His impassive eyes swept past me with metronomic precision, like a lighthouse beacon overlooking a sinking vessel beneath its cobbled walls.

Later, I would come to understand that I had expected too much of Sutton during our first meeting. After all, his job wasn't to patch me up emotionally, but to explain a tricky surgical procedure and why it was necessary. Ours was an unfortunate, even traumatic pairing, yet it had to occur. Without it there could be no beginning or future, only a past.

The days and weeks and years ahead would reveal another Leslie Sutton, a deeply caring physician who held himself up to painfully high standards and was solicitous toward anxious parents. Beneath his academic patina also was a delightful, self-deprecating wit, which bubbled to the surface during relaxed moments.

Once, years after our first encounter, I asked Sutton why brains are packed in cerebrospinal fluid, like a lowly can of tuna fish. After walking me through a few of the more popular theories, none of which has ever been proven, Sutton confessed that nobody knew. "It's a good question," he said. "And when patients ask me, I tell them it's there to provide me a living."

But as I mentioned, these insights would come later. Our first meeting was all business, with Sutton wasting no time describing the procedure he would perform—assuming we consented—to close the lesion on Cary's back.

First, Sutton explained, he would rupture the thin sac and drain the cerebrospinal fluid that had pooled there during the last few months. Then, he would unwrap the bundles of nerves and fibrous membranes that had tangled at the point of the lesion instead of extending down the spinal column to the muscles and organs nature had intended them to serve. If he happened upon any live nerves, as occasionally occurred, he would try to steer them on their way, although, Sutton hastened to add, it was unlikely it would make a difference. Most, if not all, of the nerves he sorted through would be dead. Similarly, the rugged dura and pia matter he recovered from the spinal cord would almost certainly be splayed and useless. Sutton estimated that the cutting and cleaning would take one hour. Then he would stretch Cary's skin across the lesion and suture it closed.

"The biggest risk we face is that the skin could break down or some of it could die," Sutton explained. If that occurred, he would be forced to graft donor skin over the wound. "I'm not expecting that to happen, but it could. It's a fairly large cele."

The trick was to stretch the skin across the wound without putting too much tension on it. The larger the sac, the more difficult the task. If you stretched the skin too tightly, it would either rip or adhere to the spinal cord as the child grew. Neurosurgeons refer to these adhesions as tethered cord syndrome because the scar tissue literally fastens itself to the cord, interfering with gait and bladder function and increasing the chances of scoliosis and other spinal deformities. Currently, surgery is the only available treatment, although the procedure is not without risk and results vary tremendously. A handful of neurosurgeons have taken to inserting a plastic guard between the spinal cord and the skin of newborns as a preventive measure. But this is still considered controversial. Most are using a looser closure so there is more space as the child grows.

Sutton took out a small model of the human spine and pointed to the mid-lumbar area. Cary's lesion had occurred around the second or third of the five vertebrae that make up this section of the spinal cord, he explained. If it had developed below that point, in the sacral section, there would have been less paralysis. Had it occurred higher, in the thoracic region, he would have had even less control. This is what Charney had meant earlier when he had referred to Cary as a "middle-of-the-roader."

After the operation, Sutton would follow Cary to see if he developed hydrocephalus—a potentially dangerous buildup of cerebrospinal fluid in his brain. This mysterious fluid winds through the ridges and valleys of nerve cells in the brain like a vast network of underground rivers, spilling into open spaces, known as ventricles, and forming tiny lakes, which in turn trickle here and there along the brain's blue highways, coursing a circuitous path back down the spinal cord. Surprisingly, for all of this activity, there is barely enough cerebrospinal fluid in an adult brain to fill a small glass. The estimate is 125cc, slightly less in a newborn. Even so, we produce enough of the brackish fluid—about eight ounces daily—to replenish our supply four times over the span of just twenty-four hours.

This last point is critical to understanding why the vast majority of children born with spina bifida develop hydrocephalus shortly after birth. In a normal brain, cerebrospinal fluid is manufactured and absorbed continuously, flowing from the ventricles, where it is produced, down the spine, and then back again within the casing of the brain, where it is reabsorbed into the blood and the process starts anew.

Because of a malformation of their brainstems, known as Chiari II syndrome, this pathway is blocked in children with spina bifida, resulting in an excess of cerebrospinal fluid in the brain's canals. Left untreated, hydrocephalus causes severe headaches, seizures, vomiting, and problems with vision. As fluid accumulates, it also distorts the size and shape of the head, giving it an exaggerated, horsey appearance.

Not that long ago, children with hydrocephalus were secreted away to government or private institutions, where they languished until they died. It wasn't until the late fifties that a physician named John Holter developed a plastic valve, called a shunt, that could be inserted into the brain to drain excess fluid. Holter's critical breakthrough was born out of necessity—a son with spina bifida and hydrocephalus.

Today, shunts are considered a staple in the treatment of newborns with spina bifida, which translated means *spine split in two*, or open spine. Once a buildup of cerebrospinal fluid is detected, usually within the first few days or weeks, a shunt is inserted into one of the ventricles and a thin plastic catheter is threaded under the skin into the abdominal cavity, where the excess fluid is reabsorbed into the blood stream.

It's a relatively simple procedure, surgically speaking, although Sutton was careful to point out that shunts commonly malfunction, requiring yet more surgery to make repairs or even a replacement. The data were dodgy. However, some estimates of the failure rate ran as high as 50 percent! The explanations were many and varied. Sometimes the devices were defective, and the tiny, bubble-shaped valve that controlled the flow stopped functioning. Other times, the catheters became clogged; all it took was a speck of protein. Frequently, it was a simple matter of a child outgrowing his tubing. Like a plumber making a house call, a neurosurgeon would go back in and extend the plastic tubing. At plumber's rates, of course. Some kids were known to have undergone three, four, even five shunt revisions, Sutton said, although they tended to be older and thus victims of the refining process. These days, with improved technology, multiple repairs were a little more unusual.

At the moment, Cary exhibited none of the classic signs of hydrocephalus. His ventricles were clear, and the fontenelle or soft spot in the middle of his head was spongy.

"It's still a little early to tell," Sutton reminded me. "But the law of averages says Cary will need a shunt within the first two weeks. Nearly all of the children do. If he doesn't he will be the exception."

Why the first two weeks? Why not while in the womb? In part, the answer has to do with the porous nature of the cele, which serves as an escape route for enough cerebrospinal fluid to maintain homeostasis. Once a lesion is sutured, there no longer is a place for the fluid to leak. It begins to pool in the ventricles, swelling up like a lake during a steady rain, exerting pressure on the rest of the brain. The brain becomes tense, if you will, and the way doctors detect the change is by checking the fontenelle. As the hydrocephalus becomes progressively worse, this small round spot, which is about the size of a half-dollar, hardens, until it no longer responds to touch. At this point, it's time to put in a shunt.

"We'll follow Cary carefully," Sutton said, "and once he starts to show signs, it will just be a question of when, not if. Okay?"

"Okay," I responded rotely.

"My understanding is you'll get back to Dr. Charney about the surgery?"

"I'm going to talk to my wife. Then we're going to call."

"Fine. It's not an immediate crisis. We have a little time."

"Thank you," I said, rising.

Sutton extended his hand. "We'll take care of things," he said.

Later that afternoon I took my other son, Gregory, aside and tried to explain what had happened during the last day and a half.

"There are some problems with your new brother," I began awkwardly. "He's going to have to stay in the hospital while the doctors do some things to help him. He's not going to die. But his back and his feet are hurt. The doctors had to take him from the hospital where he was born to a special hospital in Philadelphia where he can get better care. So when I take you to see him, he won't be at the same hospital with Mommy. And he will be in this contraption that looks a little bit like a fish tank. Only Cary's inside. Do you understand?"

Gregory shook his head. "Can I go and play now?" he asked.

"Not just this second. Don't you want to hear about your little brother?"

"Grammy already told me."

Alerted earlier, Cathy's mother and father had come to our house to help out while I traveled back and forth between hospitals.

"What did Grammy say?"

"I don't know," Greg fidgeted. "That Cary had a problem."

"Okay, but I was with him. Don't you want to know anything else?"

Greg looked down at his hands. He was barely five years old. How could he understand?

"Cary's not going to die," I repeated quietly. Even if Greg wasn't interested, I imagined this was the one piece of information he probably needed to know; the one question he might squirrel away in his unconscious like a seed.

"Can I go play now?"

"Yes."

Gregory popped off of the floor. His pale blue eyes were clouded, and I wondered now whether this conversation had been a mistake. "Just do me a favor," I said. "I need you to be on your best behavior for Grammy and Papa the next few days. Do you think you can do that for me?"

"Yes."

"That would be a great help to me."

Greg scooted away again to his toys. Exhausted, I lay my head against his bed and closed my eyes. Even the simplest intention seemed overly complicated now. My entire person seemed to be on overdrive, accelerating wildly, heading toward a crash who-knows-where.

Before I visited Cathy, I went for a short run along a creek near our home. I had run here hundreds of times in all kinds of weather. But now, with the light fading quickly, it looked bleaker and more austere than I remembered.

Without warning, I started to cry, first a trickle of big burning tears, then a steady stream that fogged my vision. Afraid someone would see me, I dared not stop, running on across a small bridge and then down into the protective wrap of a wooded path.

"I can do this," I suddenly heard myself say, like a student psyching himself for a test. "I can do this. I can make a good life for you, Cary. I promise you I can."

That evening I shared everything Charney and Sutton had said with Cathy. She was still groggy and in pain, but what really hurt was being separated from Cary.

"I can deal with the medical decisions," she said, stopping to catch her breath, "because they have to be made. What I can't stand is not knowing whether Cary is happy or sad or if he needs me. I see these other mothers and it feels like I didn't even give birth."

Nothing I could say could make the terrible emptiness Cathy felt go away. Only holding Cary close to her breast could do that. And yet that was still three or more days away. While time had compressed for me into a small hard ball, it had exploded around Cathy, swirling outward like a vast black hole.

Before Cathy even called Ed Charney, she had made up her mind to approve the surgery. But it was while she was on the phone that her reasoning suddenly spilled out.

"I had this feeling all along that something was wrong. I didn't know what. It just didn't feel like a normal pregnancy," she explained. "Then when Cary was born and they told us about the problems, my attitude just changed completely. I knew that we were given this special child for a reason, and that we were going to be better because of it. And when I saw him, I thought how beautiful he was. He looked like my other son, Gregory, only smaller."

Cathy had never mentioned her concerns before. Now,

I found myself at a loss. Why hadn't she shared her feelings with me? With her doctors? It would be months before I had answers to these questions.

Normally, we would have met with an anesthesiologist before Cary's surgery to hear about the various dangers of administering drugs to infants. Anticipating our decision, Charney had already arranged for Cary to be placed on the operating room schedule for the following morning, which meant one of us would have to give our consent to the anesthesiologist verbally.

"I can have him call first thing in the morning," Charney said.

"He can call me at home," I said.

"It's going to have to be early. They start around six o'clock."

"I'll be up."

Before I left, Cathy told me how earlier in the day, Dr. Milspa, one of the members of the OB–GYN practice she used, had been to visit. "He was so nice. He stayed for a long time and told me how one of his children was born with a disability, and how it was such a shock at first. But once they got the baby home, he said everything began to change. They got to know the baby and pretty soon they weren't focusing on his problems. They were treating him like just another child. Gil, it was so positive to hear someone who had been through it, I wish you could have been here."

"Me, too."

"What he said really made a difference. I stopped feeling sorry for myself. Now all I want to do is see Cary."

"You will," I said, "soon."

I slipped out of bed early the next morning and went

downstairs. What had Charney said—the anesthesiologist would call around six? A wall clock read five-thirty. It was still dark outside.

Now what? I was hungry but not hungry at the same time. Awake but still shrouded in morning's fog.

I decided to make the most of the half-hour by planting some grass seed I had been meaning to put out weeks ago. We did not have a big front yard, but I tore at it now with a rake until my arms and back ached. The conditions were ideal, cool and damp, and the old grass flew away on the metal tongues, cutting thin, neat rows for seed. A crow the size of a small dog eyed my work hungrily.

The phone rang at six-thirty-five. I caught it before the first ring had even finished. A husky voice identified itself as Dr. Shipman, the anesthesiologist. A nurse named Kim was also listening to the conversation, as a legal precaution.

"As with anything we do," Shipman began, "the administration of anesthesia to children carries a small but real risk."

Even today, years later, I cannot shake loose any more of our conversation. I know it was brief and that Shipman was helpful but abrupt. What I recall most vividly, however, is the cold, sinking sensation that began in my stomach and raced through my body, numbing it, as though I were the one about to be cut.

FOUR

The Calculus of Disease

We did not choose this experience, one which has thrown us up against the unknown and back again so many times. Few ever do. And they are saints. Or at least stronger and possessed of far greater love than most.

Our gift snuck up on us, a wispy ghost that defied all medical histories, imaging and prodding. To the best of my recollection, there was never so much as a hint of a problem, let alone blood or pain. One misty April morning we started out on one journey. Six years later, we have yet to return from another.

Now, giddy with newfound technology, a small but growing band of researchers insist that they can identify 90 percent of all fetuses with spina bifida in the womb—and do so before twenty-four weeks, the legal cutoff for abortions. I do not believe them. Not for one moment. Because they are researchers trading in a neat and tidy universe. And because I can not afford the emotion.

Still, I find myself worrying over the possibilities at odd hours. What if it is possible? What if doctors can stare inside these swollen bellies and know? And what of the surprised and fragile parents left to decide the fate of their unknown babies? How can they possibly see past their pain and make a fair decision? I wonder how many doctors will suggest they visit a family with a child born to this infuriating condition? How many will even know how to find such a family?

I have been thinking about these questions for some weeks now because I know the time is coming. I may not believe it, but I understand. For all I know, it may already be here.

Only the other day, another researcher predicted that doctors will soon be able to patch the shattered spinal cords of fetuses with spina bifida by performing surgery while they are still in their mother's womb. Using allogenic bone grafts and a paste of agar, bone, and fetal tissue, they will build these fetuses a new neural tube to encase their spinal cord and brain. At that point, nature will take over.

"It's not a terribly difficult procedure to do," explains Dr. Maria Michejda of the Georgetown University School of Medicine, as though it were no harder than working with plaster of paris. Locked in her Washington area lab, Michejda has been performing the procedure for years on damaged monkeys, with promising results, she reports.

The biggest hurdle, and the reason Michejda's work

probably hasn't received more publicity, is that it involves fetal tissue. In 1988 the Reagan administration banned federally funded research using tissue from aborted fetuses, contending it might lead to an increase in abortions. This ruling eliminated most fetal research and left physicians like Michejda, who continue to work in the area, walking on egg shells.

"It is very sensitive and I must be careful," she said during an interview. She hastened to add that she does not use tissue from elective abortions, only from spontaneously aborted fetuses. The distinction is important, if not scientifically, at least politically.

Politics aside, I find myself oddly ambivalent about Michejda's achievements. Surely her research offers reason to hope and pray. One day, it may even spare parents the shock and pain of a shattered birth. And yet, I am left with a peculiarly bitter taste in my mouth.

Why, I wonder, is medicine so accomplished at cutting and pasting, the mechanics of curing, yet so indifferent toward caring for the children already burdened with physical defects? Here, the ranks of dedicated doctors thin to a handful, attention spans wander, and the sweeping intellectual current of medicine slows to a trickle. Even more painful is the insulting manner in which these children are shuffled into the scientific equivalent of back rooms, strip-searched by inexperienced residents who poke and prod and ask the same fumbling questions over and over, providing few details and little or no insight, only to vanish like specters. Are our children nothing more than educational materials? Do they not have feelings and eyes? Do they not have lives?

Ah, but I am being unfair here. We expect too much as parents. We still dream and believe in the impossible.

Many of us have bought the curing image of medicine, despite all of our best instincts, and have yet to rinse our mouths of the acrid taste of disappointment. That, too, will come in time. For some lucky souls, it already has. Untethered, they are rising up and demanding to be heard, insisting that their children be cared for with the same attention and respect as able-bodied children. Insisting, in short, that they be treated like human beings.

Still, painful though this may be, it is not what cuts to the marrow, not what stabs at my heart. This is harder to explain and quite possibly a contradiction. It is this: while I wish our son to be free of hurt and pain, saved from ridicule and blind fear, and while I have dreamed of him throwing off the heavy braces that lock his legs, I know that were we given the choice today between the full magic of medicine and imperfection, between the son we have and another physically perfect child, we would make that choice without blinking, without qualms, and our lives would be richer for doing so.

We would choose Cary.

But none of this explains, why us? Why, out of a thousand couples, were we the ones singled out by nature to have a baby with spina bifida? What mysteries and secrets were locked away in our ragged biological pasts?

For months, Cathy and I wrestled with these questions without finding answers. We talked with genetic counselors and read materials given to us by local spina bifida groups. We even purchased medical texts searching for explanations that never seemed to be there.

In time, we would come to understand why this was the case. So little basic research had been done into the causes of spina bifida that medicine had only the most meager details to offer new parents such as ourselves. Cast into his void, we were left to fumble our way along with everybody else, drifting between anger and confusion, quietly blaming ourselves, always desperate for threads of understanding.

The simplest answer, one that we heard. frequently during our initial research, was also the most unsatisfying. The conception of a baby is a biological crap shoot, we were told, a random comingling of chromosomes and genes representing two separate and unique biological histories. Given the correct circumstances, anything is possible. The calculus of disease, mysterious and often extreme, is nearly infinite.

In some childhood illnesses, such as sickle-cell anemia, cystic fibrosis, and certain cancers, a single defective gene is the culprit. Because genes instruct our cells to create specific proteins, they control the physical traits we inherit. Sometimes all it takes is one faulty gene to unravel nature's work and cut a child down, bending limbs and weakening muscles, obstructing lungs with mucous or destroying red cells before they can feed the body with oxygen-rich blood.

Other childhood maladies—and spina bifida is a prime example—seem to involve multiple defective genes. Geneticists, for instance, estimate that upward of twenty or more genes may falter during the formation of the neural tube, the embryonic housing for the brain and spinal cord, in such children. Tracking so many genes is extraordinarily difficult. That is one reason why these children may be poor candidates for gene therapy, an emerging yet potentially revolutionary procedure in which a healthy gene is substituted for a faulty gene in hopes of taking over its function.

How and why do the genes of some fetuses misfire while other children with nearly identical profiles go unscathed? The answers vary from disease to disease and condition to condition. But as with so many other human endeavors, timing appears to be everything. Take the case of spina bifida. Although much remains to be unraveled about this mysterious condition, researchers generally agree on the following scenario.

Approximately two to five weeks following conception, during a critical stage when masses of undifferentiated cells are receiving their genetic instructions, something goes awry in a cluster of genes whose job is to direct the construction and final closure of the neural tube. Researchers speculate that either the messages from these genes never arrive at the designated cells, appear in tatters, or else show up unfashionably late, after the critical period for the formation of the neural tube has passed.

Normally at this point, approximately twenty-eight days, the neural tube zippers shut, with the embryonic brain at one end and the fledgling spinal cord at the other. In fetuses with spina bifida, the neural tube fails to close, leaving an opening where a bony fragment protrudes upward and countless neural tissues and nascent nerves tangle into a knot, instead of migrating down the spine to their intended muscles and organs. The result is paralysis below the point of interruption, although levels vary.

However, this still does not explain what triggers the faulty genes. Why one family and not another? Is it as random as we were led to believe, or is there a pattern?

The answers to these seemingly simple questions are more mysteries. All science currently can tell us is that there is not one cause of neural tube defects. Some cases appear to be part of a genetic syndrome, while others are caused by medical problems during pregnancy, such as gestational diabetes or fever. Still other cases seem to be triggered by substances in the environment, known as teratogens, the list of which comprises a veritable grab bag of medications, household chemicals, and toxic agents.

Diet is yet another culprit, especially deficiencies in zinc, iodine, ascorbic acid, and folic acid, a B vitamin found in leafy green vegetables, citrus fruit, and whole grains. The latter has attracted particular attention in Ireland and Wales, where rates of spina bifida are among the highest in the world, and local diets are known to be low in roughage containing folic acid.

Several studies during the last decade have reported sharp declines in neural tube defects after women who had previously given birth to a baby with spina bifida were placed on multivitamin therapy with folic acid supplements. However, most of these studies had been flawed in one way or another.

Then, in July 1991, British researchers published a landmark study in the medical journal *Lancet* showing that women who took 4 mg of folic acid before conception and during early pregnancy cut their chance of having a second baby with spina bifida by 72 percent.

Officials at the Federal Centers for Disease Control in Atlanta quickly embraced the finding and recommended that American women who had already given birth to a baby with the disabling condition take folic acid if they planned another pregnancy.

In September of 1992, CDC officials strengthened their recommendation, advising all women of child-bearing age to consume 0.4 milligrams of folic acid daily to reduce their chances of having a baby with neural tube defects.

The updated recommendation applies to all women and

not just those trying to become pregnant because approximately half of all pregnancies are unplanned, Dr. Godfrey Oakley of the CDC's division of birth defects and developmental disabilities said.

"This (recommendation) will save lives of some children who might otherwise have died," explained CDC Director William L. Roper. "It will also reduce the lifelong disability which other children who survive with spina bifida now experience."

The average American woman consumes about 0.2 milligrams of B vitamin folic acid daily in a regular diet, according to CDC estimates. Even if she adds a supplement or multivitamin with 0.4 milligrams to her diet, she should still be within a range considered safe by the U.S. Food and Drug Administration.

For many months, Cathy worried that she was responsible for Cary's defect. If only she had eaten a better diet or hadn't given the cat a flea dip, he would not have suffered this defect, she believed. Then, too, she had developed a mild case of diabetes during her pregnancy, and that could have caused his deformity.

I knew she was being unfair to herself. But how do you tell someone that? How do you break through their veil of pain with ordinary words? In time, I came to see these fitful bouts as part of the grieving process. Cathy had to blame someone or something. Who better, closer, and more convenient than herself?

During these first weeks and months, I took solace that we were not alone in confronting this horrendous defect. Untold families were struggling with many of the same fears and questions. And even though I did not know them, I drew strength from the common bonds we shared.

This slim, unspoken thread was enough. It helped me confront the uncertainty we faced and cut through the powerful loneliness that overwhelms parents of chronically ill and disabled children.

For a time I also permitted myself the luxury of ignorance. Spina bifida might be a capricious bullet fired blankly into a crowd, I reasoned, but at least it was democratic, striking families of all manner and kind. We might fairly wonder: Why us? But not: Why not them?

It was years before I learned differently. The bullet I knew as spina bifida wasn't really so random. In fact, it seemed to have the names of its victims printed on its narrow casing. Consider:

While spina bifida is recognized on all continents and has appeared in medical literature for thousands of years, frequency rates are significantly higher in some countries than in others. Variations also exist within countries, with certain regions hit much harder than others.

The British Isles, for instance, have the highest known rates of spina bifida and anencephaly, a related neural tube defect in which all or part of the brain is absent. Overall, approximately four out of every thousand live* births are affected. Yet in Northern Ireland and Southern Wales, the rate is closer to nine out of every thousand live births. No one can say why. Other countries with high rates include Egypt, Pakistan, India, and sections of China. Those with extremely low rates are Finland, Israel, and Japan.

In the U.S., spina bifida is most common in southern

---

*The key words here are "live births." An estimated 35 to 40 percent of all conceptions result in spontaneous loss due to a defect. Approximately ninety percent of all neural tube defects result in loss. The bottom line: birth defects are far more common than generally thought.

Appalachia. The lowest rates are in the West. Again, no one knows why. Nor can they explain why the rate of spina bifida has declined sharply during the last fifty years even as the number of people surviving with the condition has increased. Or why there has been no comparable decline in other well-nourished nations, such as New Zealand.

Another baffling question is why neural tube defects vary sharply among different ethnic groups, with lower rates among blacks, Asians, and certain groups of Jews, and higher ones among the Irish and Sikhs.

I am three-quarters Irish. Cathy is French and German. So, in theory, we would appear to be at slightly higher risk relative to the rest of the population. Yet the genetic counselors we spoke with weren't overly impressed by this information. It was one possible factor, they said, not a smoking gun.

Moreover, our family histories contained no evidence of neural tube defects. That is not unusual. Nearly 90 percent of all cases of spina bifida involve couples with no history. It is as though the condition rises up out of the pitch, the accumulation of thousands of years of genetic evolution compressed into a single moment.

It is no accident that so little is still known about the causes of spina bifida.

Although this terrifying condition dates back at least twelve thousand years, the medical community essentially ignored unlucky infants born with spina bifida until the early sixties, practicing what one doctor aptly termed "therapeutic nihilism."

Even today, many elements of American society remain profoundly indifferent. Consider that it wasn't until 1991 that the words "spina bifida" even appeared in a congressional bill authorizing spending for medical research. And try finding mention of spina bifida in the tens of thousands of pages of research findings published annually by the National Institutes of Health. I did and came away sorely disappointed.

What makes this so unnerving is that federally funded research is the lifeblood for understanding the basic science and processes of any disease. Without these dollars, it is hard to imagine anyone unraveling the mystery of spina bifida, let alone understanding how to prevent it. Yet, for the last half century, Congress and medicine's top bureaucrats have ignored the nation's most common physical birth defect. Harsh words? Absolutely. Yet words that are backed by numerous statistics.

In 1990, the NIH financed $7.3 billion worth of biomedical research through its seventeen different disease-specific centers. Of that amount, $1.6 billion went for cancer research, nearly $1.1 billion for heart research, and more than $580 million for research into diabetes and kidney diseases.

Within these broad categories, AIDS, or acquired immune deficiency syndrome, was the single biggest winner, receiving $717 million in NIH funds. Including all other sources of federal funds, AIDS research grants totaled more than $1.2 billion in 1990 and are expected to exceed $2 billion in 1992.

By way of comparison, the NIH set aside just $3.2 million dollars in 1990 for research related to spina bifida. At least that was all the money I could find in my review of NIH budgets and interviews of budget officers for the individual institutes. Some likely grantors, such as the Institute for Arthritis and Musculoskeletal Diseases, didn't spend so much as a dime on spina bifida, even though it is the number-one crippling birth defect in the U.S. Others, like the Institute of Child Health and Human Development, which had a budget of $442 million, doled out $1 million for research related to spina bifida.

The point isn't to pit cancer patients against children with spina bifida and other conditions. Nor is it to create an entitlement mentality. Indeed, one could fairly argue that precisely such an attitude has skewed research funding during recent history, opening it up to bullying, politics, and media-orchestrated pressure.

Rather, it is to illustrate how federal research funding as it is currently practiced is inequitable, shortsighted, and by its nature, a zero-sum equation. The economic law of scarce resources, remember, also applies to medical research. Congress and the NIH can't award hundreds of millions of dollars for AIDS studies without sacrificing other diseases. Without powerful lobbies and attention-grabbing spokespeople, childhood maladies like spina bifida get lost in the shuffle.

The Spina Bifida Association of America is trying, and recently it has made some headway. However, unlike some of the bigger and better-endowed disease advocacy groups, its financial resources are limited. In 1990, this Washington area nonprofit organization lost more than half a million dollars on revenues of only $1.2 million dollars, according to a copy of its public tax return. One consequence is that this grass-roots group only recently had the funds to start lobbying Congress for research grants.

Medical researchers also are nobody's fools: they follow the government money trail like everyone else. If there is no money available for a particular disease, they look to other diseases to study. And when they see the money trail shifting, they shift along with it.

In the sixties, cancer and heart disease were the hot areas. Now it's AIDS. For political and financial reasons, the trail has never veered toward children whose legs don't work, whose spines curve at horrendous angles, and whose heads swell with excess spinal fluid. We can debate why—but only up to a point. The bottom line remains that these children have usually been left off to the side somewhere, out of the klieg lights and away from the microphones, left to pity, without help or understanding.

Listen to Donald H. Reigel, a neurosurgeon who directs one of the country's largest spina bifida clinics at Allegheny General Hospital in Pittsburgh. During a visit, he related how he once searched back years at the National Institutes of Health to see what grants had been awarded for spina bifida.

"All I could find was one fifty thousand-dollar grant," he said. "This is the most common (physical) birth defect. It exerts a tremendous toll on these kids and their families. It's horrendously expensive to society. And the primary source of federal research funds has only given one fifty-thousand-dollar grant in ten years? It's a disgrace."

David McClone, a neurosurgeon at Children's Memorial Hospital in Chicago and another dedicated advocate for children with spina bifida, agrees that federal research funding has been scarce. However, he offers a more positive view of the situation, pointing out that a number of national conferences have recently examined the causes of spina bifida, resulting in a series of federal contracts to study neural tube defects in animals.

McClone notes: "A year and a half ago, absolutely nothing was going on. At least now we are talking about the problem and bringing it to the attention of Congress and policymakers. The bottom line is: dollars generate research. Without money, nothing is going to happen. We have to get some dollars. We need to make our case."

Why haven't federal health officials recognized this need on their own?

It can't be because there aren't sufficient numbers of children to justify investing in research. Federal data buttress this point. According to the Center for Disease Control, between 1980–1987, an estimated 13,600 infants in the United States were born with spina bifida, approximately one-quarter of whom subsequently died as a result of their defects.

Overall, more than one million children in America suffer from a chronic illness or physical defect so severe they require assistance with such basic activities of daily living as bathing, eating, and changing their clothes. An estimated ten million additional children suffer from less severe chronic conditions.

The cost of caring for these children is substantial. The CDC estimates that the annual cost of medical and surgical care for all persons with spina bifida exceeds $200 million. The yearly bill for all disabled and chronically ill children is more difficult to unravel. However, it is believed that in 1990 spending reached between $4 to $6 billion, surely a sufficiently large enough number to warrant more research funding.

"Children who suffer from chronic illness are a neglected group in our society," writes Harvard University pediatrician James M. Perrin, one of the nation's leading experts on the subject. Although a growing segment of the childhood population, they "have lacked serious public attention to their needs and to the heavy burdens their families bear."

The neglect extends from the formulation of coherent public policies affecting disabled children to the most basic issue of how many children are born with a birth defect each year.

When I asked a physician in the CDC's Birth Defects and Monitoring Program the latter question, he responded with an estimate of between 100,000 to 150,000 children annually, a margin of error of plus or minus 50 percent. Stunned, I looked a little closer. It turned out that the agency's vaunted system for monitoring birth defects includes data for only one-third of U.S. births annually; it excludes stillbirths; it is based on hospital medical records, which often are incomplete or wrong, and it is designed to function as a kind of early warning system, not as a precise repository of medical data.

Is it any wonder then that no one seems to know the number of children born each year with spina bifida? During my research, I came across four apparently authoritative estimates—some government, some private— ranging from a low of 1,500 to a high of 9,000.

All of which I might be able to dismiss were it not for the profound implications it holds for public policy. Simply put, if you don't how many children have severe birth defects, how do you plan to treat them, or know what financial and medical resources you will need?

The answer is, you don't. You fumble your way along. And these children slip through the cracks of a jury-rigged system. As we would discover only too well during the years ahead.

FIVE

Small Victories

Those first days passed in a blur. More than once, I caught myself signing forms without understanding what I was agreeing to or how it would affect Cary. Exhausted, I felt a spirit stir outside my body, watching down on a man moving in slow motion, bleary-eyed and numb, struggling to hold on to any props he could find.

"You need more rest," Cathy worried from her hospital bed. "You can't keep this up."

She was right, of course. But what choice did I have? Until she was released from the hospital, and felt well enough, it was my responsibility to watch over Cary and act as a courier of important news. Irrationally, I told myself that I could rest when I returned to work, over-looking the fact that my schedule would be even more crowded then. Not only would I be putting in a full day at *The Inquirer,* but I would also be traveling crosstown after work to spend the evening with Cary. The truth was I couldn't let go. My heart and my mind wouldn't allow me. Afraid of what I couldn't control, I felt an overwhelming need to protect my son, even if this only meant pulling a rocker up next to his crib. There was no reasonable explanation for such behavior. Intellectually, I understood that Cary was in good keeping; in fact, I had come to trust Marion Logue, his nurse, implicitly. Yet emotionally, I was certain that the day I skipped a visit would be the day something terrible went wrong. To make matters worse, the normal flow of hospital routine offered ample opportunity for mischief. Buried in the hurried scribblings of doctors and nurses, offhand comments and shuffling of patients were countless signals and codes meaning one thing to medical personnel, but something entirely different to parents and strangers.

Early one morning, for instance, I entered the unit to find Daniel Guo, a third-year medical student from Penn, bent over Cary's chest.

"What is it?" I politely interrupted.

Surprised, Guo pocketed his stethoscope like a thief. "I was just listening to your son's heart," he said. "Cary has a slight heart murmur."

"You're kidding."

"No. I just now heard it," Guo insisted.

I looked at the medical student cross-eyed. Handsome to a fault, Guo was a multicultural star, the offspring of an American mother and Chinese father, with jet black hair swept back in a modest ponytail, lazy brown eyes, which now avoided my own, and a rumpled wardrobe straight out of L. L. Bean catalogue.

"Are you sure? I said. "No one has said anything about a heart murmur to me."

Pressed, he quickly began to retreat, moonwalking toward a crib on the other side of the unit and fishing there for a chart. "I can mention it to one of the residents, if you'd like," he finally suggested.

"Please," I said, "if you wouldn't mind."

"Sure, before I leave."

Guo either forgot or never bothered, perhaps out of embarrassment. Later that afternoon, I asked Charlie Drayton, the senior resident attached to the unit, why I hadn't been told about Cary's heart murmur.

"What heart murmur?" he asked.

"The one Daniel Guo told me he heard this morning."

As senior resident, Drayton was responsible for keeping the unit's house in order. Rangy and affable, he managed to do so with good humor and remarkably little sleep, abilities I admired greatly. But now he found himself at a loss and turned to Marion Logue for help.

"This is the first I've heard of it," Logue shrugged, grabbing Cary's ringfolder from the bin and rapidly thumbing through the pages for a clue. "Nothing," she said after a moment, sliding the black folder over to Drayton.

"Forget that. Let's go see for ourselves," Drayton said.

Led by the senior resident, who had once been a reserve guard on his college basketball team and still had an athletic bounce to his step, a cluster of doctors-in-training and nurses descended upon Cary, one after another listening to his heart. Nothing. The alleged murmur had either gone into hiding or else didn't exist.

Chagrined, Charlie Drayton said he would have a word with Mr. Guo.

"Is it normal practice to allow medical students to wander around unsupervised?" I inquired privately.

"Yes and no," Drayton replied. "They do a rotation during their third and fourth years, sometimes earlier if they're really sharp. And as part of that, we do allow them to watch and participate, so long as it's nothing complicated. But they're not supposed to be making diagnoses, and certainly not telling parents their kid's got a new problem. That's my fault. I should have been watching Mr. Guo more closely."

"Look, I'm not mad at you," I said. And I wasn't. "It's just, I have enough to worry about without someone telling me Cary has a heart murmur."

"I understand," Drayton said. "You have a right to be upset. I'll speak to Dan."

"Tell him that parents are sensitive to this sort of thing. We're all just a little on edge," I said.

"I'll take care of it," Drayton said.

I saw Daniel Guo wandering through the unit several times after that. But he turned sheepish on me, burrowing his head in charts every time I neared, and we never had a chance to talk.

Two days after Cary was born, Leslie Sutton performed a two-hour operation to close the lesion on his back. I waited out the procedure on a wooden bench across from the surgical suites, which I couldn't help noticing were named in honor of C. Everett Koop, the famous pediatric surgeon who had first separated Siamese twins at CHOP and now served as the Surgeon General for the Reagan administration. It was the Department of Health and

Human Services, where Koop worked, that had led the charge on the Baby Jane Doe case, pitting the political power of the government against the will of the infant's parents. The irony of the moment was not lost on me. What if, I wondered once more, we had decided against this operation? Would someone at the hospital have used the government hot line to call HHS attorneys? Would they have filed legal papers to intercede? Would an essentially private matter have gone public, complete with Action Cam updates and the insectlike attention span of television reporters? I would never know.

Now I found myself battling against images from an uncharted future. What would Cary's life be like? How could he play with other children if he couldn't jump and run and ride a bike? Surely, they would notice and say things. How would he feel then? I felt my heart sinking. Hold on, hold on. What was it Ed Charney had said: You learn to take one day at a time. I was getting ahead of myself again. I had to stop, slow down, deal with what was in front of me, not years ahead. But how?

Every so often, a tall, solicitous nurse with a clipboard appeared to update the waiting parents. "Surgery has started and everything seems to be going well," I recall her telling me at one point. "Dr. Sutton has begun to close and expects to be finished soon," she said another time. I was thankful for these brief messages that broke through the wall separating me from Cary, but I was also wary of their potential for danger. Several times I'd watched with horror as parents started to shake and crumble at the news they received, and then retreated down the hallway, where they clung to each other in a knot.

Sutton appeared shortly before noon and sat down on the bench beside me. "It seemed to go well," he said. "But

I had to really work to stretch the skin. I'm a little worried whether it's going to hold."

"You'll watch it?" I said, recalling our earlier conversation.

"We'll check several times a day. I think it's going to be okay. You just never can be sure where there's such a large lesion."

Sutton did not say what he had found inside the sac and I did not ask, afraid to hear.

"We'll also be following Cary for signs of hydrocephalus now that surgery's over," Sutton explained. "If it's going to happen, we'll see it in the next couple of days. But if everything goes well, Cary can go home in another week to ten days."

I rode these hopeful words like the wind and was barely able to contain myself on the phone with Cathy. She also had some good news. Dr. Milspa, her obstetrician, had told her she would be released Thursday, less than thirty-six hours away. "If you drive me, I can visit Cary," she said hopefully.

"Are you kidding," I said, "that's great!"

That night I drove back to Children's Hospital to see Cary. It was raining, and the city was shrouded waist-high in mist as I headed up Civic Center Boulevard to the university area where CHOP is located.

A decade earlier, some industry officials had taken to calling the then-new hospital "a Taj Mahal" because of its layered architecture and spacious atrium with towering fountain and McDonald's restaurant. But on this night, filtered by slanting rain and the sulfurous pall of street lights, even CHOP lost some of its luster, its square-jaw lines and clear, bright lights fading in the gloom and grit of city weather.

The nurses' station outside Cary's unit was deserted except for a small cluster of nurses and residents huddled over patients' charts or talking quietly. Marion Logue, whom I had come think of as Cary's nurse, was there. And Drayton, who never seemed to sleep, and this evening looked it. Without pausing, I waved hello and headed inside.

When I reached Cary's isolette, I froze. The light was off and the gaggle of IV tubes and wires now hung limp from a pole. Cary was nowhere to be found.

I nearly sprinted back to the nurses' station, where a half-dozen heads popped up at once. "Where's Cary?" I demanded. "Where is my son?"

"He's there, isn't he?" Marion Logue said. She looked past me into the unit. There was a slight edge to her voice. Was it panic?

"No, he's not."

"What?"

"The isolette is empty."

A quick turn of recognition softened Logue's face. "Oh, that," she said, casually waving a hand. "We moved Cary to one of the cribs. Did you check against the windows?"

I hadn't considered the possibility.

"Come on, I'll show you," Logue said, rising off of her stool.

Sure enough, Cary was sleeping heavily in a crib along the bank of windows facing onto the boulevard. I let out a long deep breath, then began to apologize.

"That's okay. I should have told you when you came in," Logue said.

We stood over Cary like two sentries. "I guess this is a

step in the right direction, isn't it?" I said after several moments.

"Cary's just doing super," Marion said. "He's a real trooper. And I'll tell you what, he sure does like to eat. This afternoon he drank a whole bottle of the frozen milk you brought over and another three and a half ounces of regular formula. I thought he was going to burst."

"He must take after me. I'm a bottomless pit."

Marion eyed my skinny profile. "Whoever, it's good, because he needs his strength."

That night I watched Cary sleep for several hours. The rain beat coldly against the unit's windows the entire time. But it didn't matter. We were safe here together. Lucky, too, to have had so many small victories in one day. I was thankful more than ever for the kindness of strangers.

Two days after Cary's surgery, Leslie Sutton dropped by the unit to inform me that Cary appeared to be developing hydrocephalus.

"It's still a little early to tell for sure, but the signs are not great," he said. "We'll probably do a scan later today or tomorrow and then make a decision."

I tried my best to shake off the news. What was the figure Sutton had said—eighty to ninety percent of children with spina bifida require a shunt? Viewed in that context, this was a normal development. No big deal.

Sutton was followed by Richard Davidson, an enterprising young orthopedic surgeon who took care of many of the children with spina bifida.

"Basically, at this point, what we are talking about is taking care of Cary's clubfeet," Davidson explained. "If he is ever going to walk, and Dr. Charney told me he looks to be a good candidate, we have to straighten his feet so they are in a weight-bearing position. Right now, they are twisting inward and down, instead of pointing ahead the way they should. The other problem is that Cary's heel cords are extremely rigid, which prevents his feet from assuming a natural position."

"How do you fix that?" I wondered.

"Good question. Essentially, what we do is release the tendons and drop his heel back down so his foot is in a natural plantigrade position. Then we place a pin in there to hold it."

"When?"

"Probably when Cary is around three months, or else thirteen pounds, whichever comes first. How much does he weigh now?"

I had to think. In all of the confusion, I couldn't recall if anyone had told us. "I think he's seven pounds," I fumbled, "seven something."

"You have time," Davidson said. "What we'll do in the interim is start casting Cary to see if we get any correction. Occasionally, a child will correct all on his own, although, to be honest, I don't think you should get your hopes up. Most of the time, we lose the correction after the casts are removed. The feet drift back in because there's nothing to hold the correction." Davidson let out an exaggerated little sigh. "And that's why we have to operate."

When he was busy, as he was now, sandwiching consultations between cases in the OR, Davidson rarely sat. He straddled the room like one of the big cats at the Philadelphia Zoo, nervously roaming between the cribs and the doorway. It was Cathy who pointed out, not in a mean-spirited way, that Davidson taught her how important it was for parents to position themselves between doctors and doorways, blocking off their escape routes until all of your questions were answered. Then, and only then, should you move.

None of which was meant to be unduly critical of Davidson. From the perspective of a busy surgeon, I'm sure his behavior was perfectly normal. Between surgery, consults, paperwork, and meetings, he was swamped. If he lingered too long, nothing would get done.

Parents, on the other hand, expected time. Surgery wasn't a job to them. It was a singularly threatening event in the lives of their children. Emotion was involved. They had everything to lose and only a little to gain. What did the surgeon have at stake? If he was successful, it was another notch in his professional belt. If he failed? Well, it was unfortunate, but there was always another case. He didn't live the failure or share the grief. That was the burden of the patient and family alone.

"Unless something happens, I'll start casting tomorrow," Davidson said, slipping toward the door. He had folded his arms, Indian-chief style, across his chest, and seemed bigger than before, almost chunky.

"Okay," I mouthed, for the moment powerless.

"We'll hope for the best."

What else could we do?

Cathy was discharged around noon on Thursday. After stopping briefly at home, which some of the neighbors had kindly decorated with blue balloons, we drove to Children's Hospital. It was an emotional ride all the way around. I was happy to have my wife back but worried because Cathy was still in a good deal of pain. She, on the other hand, was anxious to see Cary after what had seemed like months, not days, but was nervous that this separation had somehow damaged their relationship. In the hallway leading to Cary's unit, we had to stop so she could catch her breath.

"Gil, I don't think I can do this," Cathy said, covering her face with her hands. "I'm so afraid."

"It's okay. You'll be fine," I tried to reassure her.

"I can't. I can't," she sobbed.

Cathy couldn't have been more wrong. Cary seemed to recognize his mom immediately, fixing on her with his luminous blue eyes and holding on. When it was time to eat, he nuzzled comfortably against Cathy and knew just what to do. Later, when Cary was sleeping, Cathy pulled up a rocking chair and studied her new son. "You know, he doesn't really look like Gregory after all," she said, turning to me. "He looks like himself." There were tears of happiness in the corners of her eyes, and I knew just what she meant.

During the drive back home, we talked openly about our fears. Up until now, these dark images had been a private matter, but now, together they spilled out in painful bursts, as though a tourniquet had been removed.

Our minds raced furiously ahead. What about school? Would Cary have to attend special schools all of his life, or would he be welcomed in the regular schools? Would he be able to keep up academically, participate in school events, take gym? And later on, would he be able to attend college, find a decent job, get married, and have a family of his own?

So little was explained, so little certain. It was wrong, thinking like this, but we couldn't help ourselves. We were living on nerves, one moment blindly optimistic, the next terrified by the unknown. We fought back tears as long as we could. But when they came, we wept openly and fully, for Cary and for ourselves.

*   *   *

On Sunday, Ronald Bowser, a pediatric fellow who was apprenticing with Sutton, advised us that an ultrasound taken earlier in the day had confirmed that Cary's ventricles were now bulging with excess cerebrospinal fluid. Without a shunt, the pressure would become unmanageable and start to wreak havoc with his brain.

"I think Dr. Sutton would like to schedule Cary for tomorrow morning," Bowser said, "unless there's a problem."

"I can't think of anything," I said.

"The procedure is fairly straightforward and only takes about twenty minutes," Bowser explained. "We make a small incision behind the right ear and insert the shunt, which is actually two tiny plastic bubbles where the fluid pools, and then we make another small incision in the abdomen to bring down the tubing to the peritoneal sac, where the fluid drains. As with anything foreign you put into the body, there's always a risk of infection or rejection. But ordinarily the biggest problem we see is shunt failure. A speck of protein gets in there and it stops working. As parents, that's what you have to watch out for. The nurses will give you information before Cary goes home that spells out the symptoms. It's pretty basic stuff—nausea, severe headaches, a sudden change in personality, irritability, an active kid who suddenly doesn't want to do anything, things like that. You'll know something is wrong. Cary just won't be himself."

In real life, of course, it's never quite so simple or easy.

Once, when Cary was eleven months old, we were worried that the shunt was failing and made an emergency visit to St. Christopher's Hospital for Children, where Cary was then being followed. Dr. Raymond Truex tested the shunt by inserting a contrast agent and tracking it down the thin tubing to Cary's stomach. It turned out it was fine. Cary had a virus that mimicked many of the symptoms of shunt failure.

"It's a common mistake. Even for some of us with extensive training, it's sometimes hard to tell the difference," Truex said.

Another time, when Cary was about two months old and we were vacationing at the beach, we noticed that his soft spot had collapsed, leaving a one-inch-wide dent in the top of our son's fuzzy head.

Alarmed, we debated what to do. On the one hand, Cary seemed fine. He was cooing happily in his chair, his eyes were clear, and he had an appetite. On the other hand, his shunt might be broken and we didn't know it. He might even be in danger.

Cathy said we should call the doctor. I was more cautious. Maybe we should wait, I suggested, and see what happens. No, we needed to call, Cathy insisted. We began to argue.

"Why are you so afraid?" I said.

"I've got a two-month-old child with something happening to him I've never seen before. I'm hours away from the nearest hospital or doctor. I think I have a *right* to be afraid," Cathy shouted.

She was right, but I couldn't admit that to myself in the heat of our argument. It was my style—and shortcoming—to try to smooth over problems in hopes that they would pass.

We marched to a phone booth across the street from where we were staying. The phone didn't work. More heated words were exchanged. We found another phone. Cathy clutched Cary to her hip while I tried to comfort

Gregory, who had picked up on our roiled emotions and was afraid. Finally, after what seemed like hours but was in fact only a few minutes, one of our pediatricians returned our call. I explained the symptoms. It didn't sound like a shunt failure, Dr. Kaltenbach said, because the symptoms were backward. The soft spot should be bulging if fluid was building up inside the brain, not depressed.

Cathy was still uncertain. If it wasn't the shunt, she said, then what was it?

"Do you want me to call the hospital?" I asked.

She nodded.

I got through to Lynn Carey-Wright, a resident in neurosurgery whom we had met previously at St. Christopher's. "Was it hot at the beach today?" she asked.

"In the mid-eighties and dry," I replied, immediately sensing where she was heading.

"Cary's probably a little dehydrated. Why don't you try giving him more to drink before you put him down for the night. As long as he's not fussing, I don't think you need to worry. On the other hand, if you need me, I'll be on call all night."

Cary slurped down a bottle and retired to his port-a-crib without complaint. The next morning we awakened to the plaintive cries of seagulls and hissing waves. We immediately went to check on Cary. Other than being hungry, he was happy as a clam. There was still a small dent in his skull, but it was much less than the previous evening. It seemed Dr. Carey-Wright was right. All he needed was a good drink.

This frightening episode taught us several valuable lessons, not the least of which was that we had to do a better job of communicating—especially me. Emotions were backed up inside us like rainwater before a sudden, violent storm. All it took was a shift in the wind to unleash them. Trapped in these swirling eddies and whirlpools, we could be dragged under before we knew it, or could even call for help.

SIX

Routines

In the months following Cary's discharge from the hospital, we fumbled our way along in ignorance and blind hope, searching for signs that our son was a normal child. The fact that Cary looked and acted like any other newborn, except for his casts and scars, helped to feed our illusions. Then, too, he was bright and cheerful and quick at tasks requiring a good memory.

Most parents want their children to excel, or failing that, to fit comfortably into the background of family and neighborhood life, making friends, succeeding at school, and eventually advancing in work and life.

We were no different in this regard. Cary's birth had

been a traumatic experience. But now that we had him back home, we were hopeful that our lives would settle back into a routine and Cary would thrive. Why not? Except for the interruptions of doctor visits and home care, we did not envision any dramatic changes in our lives. We shared most of the same hopes and aspirations that we had for Greg. We certainly didn't anticipate that Cary's condition would steal away a sizable chunk of his childhood. We simply wouldn't allow such a thing.

How could we have known otherwise? We had nothing to compare Cary's condition against, no history, no context, no emotional background. That would come later, after years of trying to beat back the disruptive force of chronic illness, and discovering this was like trying to stop the ocean's advance by building a wall of sand. The waves of exhaustion and pain and sadness that crashed onto our lives eventually found their way into every nook and cranny of our spirits.

"A chronic illness is a constant and sometimes overwhelming companion, a shadow both inseparable and eternal," writes Robert K. Massie, Jr., a former chaplain at Yale New Haven Hospital and hemophiliac, whose story was told by his author-parents, Robert and Suzanne Massie, in the book *Journey*.

Statistics tell us that it has the power to darken and kill, as witnessed by the alarmingly high rates of depression and suicide among the disabled, more than twice the national average. But even among the emotionally healthy, a chronic condition or severe disability dominates life, weaving its insidious path into the most basic everyday experiences. Dressing. Bathing. Grooming. Going to the bathroom. Getting to and from work, assuming there is a job available. Shopping. Cooking. The able-bodied person doesn't think twice about these routines. But to an adult with spina bifida, they represent major undertakings, requiring extra time, planning, and help. It isn't surprising then that the condition or illness is frequently inseparable from the person. Viewed this way, a chronic disease or physical malformation is a tyrant, seizing one's past, present, and future and holding them hostage. Like a schoolyard bully, it demands payment and recognition. Those who ignore its warnings do so at their own risk.

And yet, it is one of life's stark contradictions that the humbling power of severe disability can also teach, nurture, and even enrich, stripping away the social detritus and shameful posturing that so often pass for knowledge and experience, to expose the authentic, unheroic self.

Life, I am reminded watching Cary, isn't made up of exclamations so much as a succession of small moments strung together like beads on a necklace. Where we go wrong is by expecting too much. Then, disappointed and empty, we have to find someone to blame. Accusations fly like personal warheads. The next thing you know it's off to divorce court! Why is it so hard to accept that life is lived in increments, not Hallmark moments? Viewed through the binoculars of experience, life is smaller, but also more sharply focused, revealing, detailed. One learns to appreciate subtle pauses in the wind, the sweep of good friends, the richness of gathered days.

Early on, we were too raw to understand these lessons. Wavering between desperate ignorance and unbridled confidence, we clung to hopeful signs wherever we found them, brushing away the danger signals. What knowledge we gleaned came later, after stumbling too many times to recount.

*   *   *

In the beginning, there was no reason to believe Cary wouldn't overcome his inital setbacks and flourish. He continued to eat well and put on weight in the weeks and months after he left the hospital. Awake between feedings, he played happily with his parents or entertained himself in his crib. At night, he slept for six hours at a stretch, allowing us well-needed sleep.

Cary, we quickly discovered, was a remarkably curious and determined baby who practiced sounds and shapes until he had committed them to memory. Upon waking, we would often find him quietly studying the bright green and red rectangular patches in a nearby quilt or busily probing the buttons and stitching of one of his many stuffed animals. His appetite for details went well beyond that of most infants and, in many ways, remains advanced today. Before the age of two, Cary taught himself the entire alphabet, upper case and lower case, and recognized all of the letters on sight. Counting and telling time followed in rapid succession. By four, he had memorized several of his favorite books and could read them by sight. Less than a year later, he could read for real. And not just beginner's books. More than once, he astounded us by nearly flawlessly reciting a page in a magazine, the television schedule in the newspaper, or a billboard along the highway. But what is truly remarkable is that he taught himself. Oh, we read to him at bedtime, and helped him sound out words, but it was Cary who strung the sounds and syllables together all by himself.

We delighted in these displays of precociousness. Perhaps Cary would compensate for his physical disabilities by being a quick and facile learner, we reasoned, repeating a favorite old saw about the disabled. Family and friends reinforced this prayer by remarking how well Cary was doing. With hindsight, it's easy to see how we were fooled. When a child can count by tens at the age of three, that's bound to impress most adults. When he sits on his bed and reads a Dr. Seuss book to himself, it's hard not to allow one's mind to wander blissfully ahead. When a toddler looks at your watch and tells you what time it is, well, that's special.

Our new son also proved to be a happy, contented baby, who eagerly engaged the world with sparkling blue eyes and a full round smile. Even on our roughest days, Cary showed us it was possible to forget the litany of medical concerns and enjoy our roles as parents. How we reveled and clung to these precious moments. How they nourished and steeled us against the tougher times, when one or another problem loomed before us like an impending storm. It was as though Cary understood we were struggling and chose these moments to be especially cute or to break out some new trick of his. One morning when I was feeling particularly sad, Cary decided to play a trick on me. I was sure he was awake because I heard him cooing and banging around in his crib while I was dressing. But when I poked my head into his room, Cary appeared to be sleeping. Moments later, I heard him rattling one of his stuffed bears against the crib rails. We went back and forth like this—me popping my head into the room and Cary pretending to be asleep, and then Cary making a racket— until we both were reduced to belly laughter.

Cary has held on to his sense of humor, playfulness, and natural curiosity about the people and things around him. In fact, he probably is a little too friendly, which occasionally causes other problems. He doesn't hesitate, for instance, to greet complete strangers and engage them in detailed conversations. Most of these people are charmed. But once in a while an encounter proves embarrassing, such as the time when our three-year-old Cary asked the woman behind us in the checkout line about her husband only to discover she was recently divorced.

"Divorced," Cary said, tossing around this idea in his mind, "Hmmmm, lady, your husband's going to be mad at you."

The poor woman turned the color of a red pepper. Outside, I advised my little interrogator that there were subjects that were off limits, including asking strangers about their husbands or wives. "Do you understand?"

"Get it, got it," Cary said, pulling out one of our standby responses to troublesome situations.

"Okay, now march."

"Divorced?" I heard Cary whisper to himself. "Are you crazy?"

Cathy was sitting on our front steps one sticky afternoon the summer following Cary's birth when a girlfriend and another woman walked by our house with their kids.

"Let me go get Cary," she said, retreating inside to collect the baby.

When she returned a minute or two later, the other woman eyed the tiny casts on Cary's feet and blurted, "What the hell happened to him?"

Gritting her teeth, Cathy replied, "He was born with clubfeet."

The stranger realized her gaffe and began to apologize. "Oh, of course, clubfeet," she sputtered. "I should have known that. My brother's one twin was born with clubfeet. They put casts on. Oh, I feel so stupid."

"No problem," Cathy said in as cheery a voice as she could muster.

The woman fidgeted, pawing at her own kids. "So," she finally chirped, "I guess we ought to be moving on now."

Because disabled children often look different—whether they are born with congenital deformities, scarred from multiple surgeries, or dependent on braces, crutches, and other appliances—they stand out in a crowd. This makes for interesting and sometimes painful encounters like the one with the thoughtless woman.

Until we moved when Cary was four, we did our food shopping at an ACME supermarket two blocks from our home. We never hesitated to bring Cary along, and he seemed to love all the activity, colors, and shapes, chattering to himself the entire time. Because of his casts, however, other shoppers seemed to feel the need to say something kind or inspirational.

"Don't worry, dear," one elderly woman advised Cathy, "God takes care of the little children. He'll be just fine."

"You know, special children all have some kind of gift," another woman counseled us. "Your son will be gifted, too."

These commentators were well meaning, of course. But the novelty of being singled out wore off quickly.

"I can't tell you the number of times I have been tapped on the shoulder by some blue-haired grandmother," Cathy marveled one evening. "It's like when you're pregnant. People seem to think you're community property because you look different."

The tone but not the frequency of the comments changed when I took Cary shopping on Saturday mornings. Early on, I noticed that there was a correlation between the age of the commentators and their faith in medicine. The older they appeared, the more persuaded they were that a miracle was just around the corner.

"You know, medicine is making wonderful progress today," a woman wearing a leopard-skinned hat exhorted me one snowy Saturday. "Doctors are discovering cures for all kinds of things. Have they found a cure for your son's feet yet?"

"I'm afraid not yet," I replied, for some perverse reason feeling a need to respond honestly. "There is no cure for clubfeet."

The poor woman didn't know what to think. Her heavily pancaked face wrinkled like tissue paper as she attempted to process this disturbing news. "I'm sorry," she said, fumbling with her purse. "I'll say a prayer for you."

Mentally, I kicked myself for being such a curmudgeon. Why couldn't I leave well enough alone, fudge the truth a little, and allow these ladies their innocent view of the world? What harm did it do?

A year or two later, when Cary began to walk with braces and crutches, our shopping trips became even more challenging. Suddenly, Cary was a "brave" and "wonderful little boy" for overcoming his disabling condition. The word "hero" began to crop up in conversation, much to our embarrassment, as in, "Hey, Dad, you've got yourself a real hero there. Keep it up. He's doing a terrific job," which is what one burly gentleman practically shouted at me. Talk about setting someone up. I felt like the father of the winning pitcher in the Little League World Series, not your run-of-the-mill dad out buying some groceries with his son.

At the other extreme were shoppers who felt an overwhelming need to help this "stricken child." At least half a dozen times we were approached by someone offering us money. "Here, this is for your little boy," they would typically say. "It's not much, but I would like you to have it."

I can't say with certainty who was more embarrassed, me, or the people trying to give us the money.

"No, no, no," I said, gently pushing the money away. "Thank you. I appreciate your generosity. But we don't need money. We're doing fine. Thank you."

A few persisted, even arguing, in which case, I offered a final "Thank you," and hurried Cary to our car.

I know these people meant well. What they didn't understand was that their comments and actions reinforced all of society's worst stereotypes of the disabled, condensing their lives into a one-dimensional world in which they were either pitiful victims who required handouts or superheroes who succeeded against all odds. Shoehorned between a rock and a hard place, there was no middle ground of experience, no tolerance for ordinariness. It was as though we were expected to live our lives as a Special Olympics production.

Parents of disabled children have a hard enough time deciding when it is appropriate to protect their children from the cruel realities of the world and when they are being overprotective. If our feelings are at all typical, these parents don't want their children viewed as victims; they don't want to cringe every time a "Miracle Telethon" is on TV, or a picture of a poster child meeting the President appears in the newspaper. These celebrity-oriented appeals may satisfy some deep-seated societal expression of pity and raise millions for publicity and research. Yet as far as we are concerned, they come at an unacceptable price.

They transform our children into tokens of tragedy, cheapening their individual worth, and denying their potential. Nor do we see our children as heroes because they learn to live with their conditions. The reality is that they muddle along like all kids, taking a detour here and a shortcut there. There may be a few—or even a lot—more detours. But that does not change the fact that they are kids. They have all of the same quirks, attitudes, and problems of other children. What they don't seem to have is superhuman powers. So please don't set them up for failure. It's difficult enough as it is. Let these children be themselves.

We struggled during these first months and years to maintain a sense of normalcy, following as many of our familiar routines as possible and inventing new ones as we went along. Sometimes our efforts worked and sometimes they didn't. But we knew it was important to try, for Cary and for the rest of the family, because to fail would have reduced our lives to a cliché. We did not want to take on the role of the wounded and special family battling against all odds; nor did we wish to see our family come apart at the seams from the stress and demands of caring for a disabled child. All we wanted was to get on with the business of living.

We went to the beach, to the amusement park, to the zoo and to the aquarium, on day trips and overnight trips. We practiced walking in the malls and anyplace else that had flat surfaces. We went food shopping, exploring in the woods, on train rides, and even down a water slide! We did things alone and together. We worked. We played. We prayed. We continued to have parties and to invite friends to our house. We went to the movies and out to eat. And once Cathy and I even got away by ourselves for a week to celebrate our tenth anniversary. It was a refreshing and long overdue break. But more important, it was a statement that we had a life apart from our children, from the caregiving and from the condition that occasionally threatened to swallow us whole.

I know that it was easier for me to adjust because I had *The Inquirer* and work to escape to each day. I might have to change my schedule, straighten out insurance problems, or take a day off here and there to attend an important medical conference, but these were relatively small interruptions compared with the day-to-day responsibilities Cathy faced at home as the primary caregiver.

This was especially the case during the first year when Cathy seemed to be running to a doctor or hospital visit every day, and sometimes two or even three times daily. Somehow, she managed to juggle her many and varied duties as mother of a busy kindergartner and infant with remarkable skill and grace, so that, to an outsider, our lives probably appeared to function like a well-oiled engine. That wasn't exactly right, of course, because Cathy was only human and suffered shortcomings like the rest of us. Her chores exhausted her. She got depressed and angry. And there were times when she resented the intrusion, and didn't hesitate to tell me.

"I know you're not given anything more than you can handle," she exploded one evening. "What I don't understand is why me? Why was *I* the one?"

What could I tell my wife? That there was no rational explanation. That it was an accident of nature, which was true. That she should not have to go through life without an explanation. Unfortunately, none of these truths helped. And so I told her what I knew.

"Why were you given Cary? Because you are strong and

practical and more creative than most women—that is why. Because no one knows the strength they have until they are taxed. And because Cary will teach you things about yourself you never knew. One day, he will help you forget the past so you can live in the present. So you can dream the future again."

If I could not help, Connie Barry usually could. Connie was Cathy's best friend in the neighborhood, a strong, loyal companion with a flashing wit and a remarkable gift for defusing difficult situations before they became truly dangerous. "Don't sweat the small stuff," Connie was fond of saying, because there was bound to be something more serious around the bend.

More often than not, it was advice from Connie that helped Cathy pull herself out of a prolonged funk, or that placed some nettlesome event in its proper perspective. For a time, another mother in the neighborhood was getting on Cathy's nerves because all she did was brag about her children. "She'll come by and if I happen to mention that Cary's done something, well, she's got to mention that her little darlings have have done that and ten other things as well."

Cathy knew that she shouldn't pay attention to the woman. But for some reason she couldn't shake the painful game of one-upmanship. Connie's blunt assessment one day finally broke her emotional logjam.

"The poor woman doesn't seem to have anything better to do," Connie said. "She's living her life through her kids and she's taking it out on you."

"I know that," Cathy said. "But sometimes I can't help it. I find myself getting caught up in her games and later I get so angry at myself for not being stronger."

"Yeah, but think of it this way. It's not fair to Cary. Why should he have to compete against her precious little ones?"

"He shouldn't."

"Well, then."

The nice thing about Connie was that she was sympathetic without being patronizing or resorting to charitable bromides. She understood we had been dealt a difficult hand, but also that we needed to get on with our lives. She didn't look upon us as victims. We were just the Gauls to her—someone to visit and share with, friends, parents, neighbors.

Our kids played together, jousted verbally, competed and battled from time to time. Connie took it all in stride. It was all part of growing up. She had come from a large, rambunctious family, so she was used to the commotion, outbursts, and tears. "What the heck," she said, "you've got to let them go crazy sometimes."

Connie always seemed to be there when we needed her. She welcomed Greg when we had to go to the hospital. She baby-sat Cary when Cathy had to go to a school conference during the day. She came to our parties and invited us back to hers. And when Cathy was feeling especially tired or down, Connie always had a cup of tea ready and some sage or funny piece of advice.

Years later, when Connie and her lawyer-husband Frank moved to Cape May, about two hours away, it was a blow. Cathy and Connie still talked on the phone and visited occasionally. But it wasn't the same. Some days I would come home from work and find Cathy sitting sadly in our kitchen. When I asked what was wrong, she would simply say, "I miss Connie." I knew what she meant.

SEVEN

Medicine Men

John Tedeschi looked at Cathy and said, "I don't know what's going to happen now."

Cathy took a deep breath. "I know," she said. "Neither do I."

Tedeschi, a man we had grown to admire and trust during the five years he had taken care of Gregory, was about to give Cary his first shot, an immunization for diphtheria, pertussis, and tetanus, or DPT for short. The needle would be delivered in Cary's upper thigh where the quadricep muscle looped into his groin.

For most parents, this would be a fairly routine event.

But to us it was more than just a shot, it was also a test of our hopes and dreams.

Eleven weeks after Cary's birth, we still didn't know if he had sensation below his waist. If Cary didn't feel this needle, it would mean the nerves serving the bulky quadricep muscles in his upper legs had been enervated. Without stimulation, they would weaken and atrophy, dimming his prospects of walking, even with the aid of braces.

Against our better judgment, we had anticipated this moment by searching for signs that Cary had feeling. It didn't matter how large or small the clue, we greedily accepted each morsel of evidence. A look of surprise when Cathy accidentally spilled a few drops of ice water on Cary's thigh was reason for hope. So, too, a leg kick on the changing table or bent knees when removing a diaper. All counted. In time, were stitched together an impressive list of otherwise random events into a convincing record. Not only would Cary walk, we had come to believe, he would be a strong walker.

Now, in the simple delivery of a needle, an event that is repeated routinely 11.5 million times each year for American children between the ages of three months and five years, our jury-rigged dream stood the risk of being dashed to pieces.

Tedeschi steadied the needle above Cary's thigh, repeating quietly, "I don't know if he's going to feel this."

Cathy struggled with whether to watch or look away. She hated needles as it was. But she was especially terrified of this one.

Tedeschi pulled back his arm. There! The needle was into the muscle and back out again in one seamless motion.

Cathy and Tedeschi stared at the baby. Nothing. Cary

gazed back at them with moon-pie eyes. Then, like a storm rushing against a clear blue day, those eyes suddenly clouded over, and Cary's pink, round face wrinkled up. His leg jerked back in protest as his first wails broke the heavy silence.

"I never thought I would say I enjoyed giving a needle, but this time I did," Tedeschi said, smiling with relief.

Cathy let out a deep sigh. "He can feel it," she said excitedly.

Tedeschi shook his head in wonderment. Then in a gesture that gently reinforced the bond between doctor and parent, he handed Cary back over to Cathy to comfort. For the moment, we could hold on to our dreams.

We were lucky to have John Tedeschi as our pediatrician. Besides being a competent doctor, John listened to our concerns, guided us when we needed direction, and was refreshingly candid in his opinions of other medical providers.

"I don't like Dr. So-and-so," he might say in a discussion of orthopedic surgeons, "His results aren't like they should be. If it were me, I would shy away from him." Or, when asked about another surgeon, "He's top-notch, really super. I've been impressed with his work. The only question I would have is how many kids with spina bifida does he treat? They're just starting up over there. So it may not be that many."

We didn't always agree with Dr. T, which is how our kids referred to John. But we appreciated his honesty. He could just as easily have been noncommittal, or have given everyone high grades, which is what happens all too often in the clubby backrooms of medicine.

We stumbled upon John Tedeschi's burgeoning group practice shortly after I joined *The Inquirer* in 1983. Cathy had heard good things about him and his then-three-member group through the mothers' grapevine in South Jersey. It just so happened that they participated in a new HMO I had selected as our health plan through work. So we decided to give the group a try.

The waiting room in the group's suburban office was packed the brisk Saturday morning we appeared for Gregory's checkup. Parents were backed up into an alcove. The phone rang constantly. Nurses hustled in and out summoning children. "This place is either incredibly popular or a mill," I whispered to Cathy.

When our turn came, we were directed to a small examining room down a horseshoe-shaped hallway. A minute or two later, a short but striking figure dressed in a lab coat, with reading glasses pushed down on the bridge of his nose, entered. "Hi, I'm John Tedeschi," he said, extending a hand first to Cathy, then to me. "And this must be Gregory. What a handsome guy."

At three, Gregory was bigger and stronger than most boys his age, with blond hair, blue eyes, and a pouty smile. Now blushing, he clung to his mom's leg and peeked at this strange new doctor with dark, wavy hair and continental good looks.

"Oh look, Mom, he's shy," John said, folding his arms.

Gregory grinned, pleased by the attention. He stepped away from Cathy and pretended to blast Tedeschi with a laser gun.

"Got me," Dr. T said, smiling.

John was remarkably gentle and friendly, which helped explain why his practice was one of the busiest in southern New Jersey. He treated all children like stars, but seemed to have a special affinity for Greg, whom he routinely referred to as "all boy."

"I could go in there ready to sell the child, but I always come out thinking he's a saint," Cathy joked.

Like anyone with good people skills, John had a bit of the salesman in him. His quiet, sensitive manner also belied a sharp mind for business and a politically seasoned practitioner. Now in his early fifties, John had watched a lot of medicine in the area and knew where many of the skeletons were hidden. But despite all of the battles and changes, he had never grown cynical or distant. In an era of high-tech medicine, he had remained a hands-on physician. He took time to chat and answer questions, no matter how innocent or desperate. Above all, he seemed to understand that there was no substitute for the age-old quality of caring.

After Cary was born, John offered us two of the most important pieces of advice we were given.

"Whatever you do," he told Cathy during one of her early visits with Cary, "don't forget Gregory. Set aside days just for him so he knows that he's still special. It's inevitable that with all of the running around you're going to be doing with Cary, Greg's time is going to get cut into. There's just so much you're able to do, right? What you don't want is for him to start to feel resentful and jealous because of his brother's illness. He needs to know he's important, too."

To me, John pointed out the importance of asking questions. "If you're not sure about something or happy with the way something is going, you have to demand that the doctors listen to you until they hear what you're saying. You're the ones living with this. In time, you'll know as much or more about Cary's condition as they do.

It will be up to you to make sure they're doing everything that needs to be done. If a doctor says Cary's going to need a renal X-ray in six months, you have to be the one to remind him, because more often than not, he'll forget. Unfortunately, a lot of this is going to fall on your shoulders. You're going to have to be strong."

We took this advice to heart, setting aside special days when Greg could choose to do anything he wanted. A bright, sensitive child, Greg was aware of the burden caring for Cary exerted on our family and the way it interfered with his young life. Many times he ended up being dragged along to Dr. T's, the hospital, or a brace shop because there was no one who could watch him. At home, we always seemed to be telling him, "Just a minute, I'm doing something with Cary, then I'll be right there. All of these minutes added up, and try as we might, we could never make them up. In this way, a disabling condition sets the agenda for all of the family members, including siblings, hovering over their days like a cloud.

Because they were five years apart in age, Greg and Cary weren't natural playmates. But they did play together, especially when Cary was a little older and could verbalize his needs, and in their own special way they watched out for each other as only brothers can do. Cary absolutely adored his older brother, whom he called "Gaggi," and followed him everywhere. If Greg was playing a video game, Cary would sit in the background and watch him. If Greg went upstairs to his room, Cary would crawl up the steps and appear in Greg's doorway. Later on, they played video games together and shared a room for a year—at Greg's invitation. Greg teased Cary unmercifully at times and blamed his brother for just about everything, but he could also be incredibly sweet and protective, especially if another kid was giving Cary a hard time.

Once, while we were riding somewhere, I asked Greg whether he ever resented having a brother with spina bifida.

"Not really," he said without hesitation. "It's no big deal. I mean we're still brothers. It's just Cary has spina bifida."

"It does get in the way sometimes," I suggested.

"That's true. But so does Little League."

The next time the boys are screaming at each other, I will try to remember that conversation. And the advice from John Tedeschi about paying attention to each of our children's needs. Dr. T's words helped to prepare us for the difficult times ahead. For that we are grateful.

Unfortunately, the John Tedeschis of the medical world were few and far between.

One of the great myths cultivated by American medicine is that all doctors are created equal. Needless to say, this is no more possible than all auto mechanics or all writers being equal. Yet even today, with the halls of medicine under attack from many different fronts, the profession persists in painting a Norman Rockwell–like image of its masters as uniformly kindly, caring, and involved.

As parents, it is difficult to give up the heroic image of the physician. We have been conditioned to believe it is fact. More important, we want it to be true. We want to turn our children over to the doctors and have them returned healed, relieving us and them of the terrible burden of imperfection. Yet, if we are to navigate the long course of a chronic illness or disabling condition without it swallowing us whole, we have little choice but to abandon the image. To do otherwise is to live a lie and open oneself to constant pain and disappointment. It is equally damaging to relegate oneself to the role of supplicant and nonparticipant in this all-consuming event. By accepting the frailties and shortcomings of physicians, it is possible to open a dialogue based on honesty and trust, in which each side views the other as partners instead of as adversaries, objects, or heroes.

Of course, getting to this stage is easier said than done. We, too, once believed, hoping against hope that our doctors show us the way. It was only much later, after many disappointments, that we came to understand and accept the imperfections of medicine, and to realize that no superstar-physician could undo what nature had done. The fundamental difference between an acute illness and a chronic disability is that one must live the disability. Even the most talented doctors cannot do that for you.

The best parents can hope for is to strike a balance between the needs of their children and the needs of their physicians. Unfortunately, these are not always the same. Parents want information, counseling, and help managing day-to-day issues, such as dealing with a child's incontinence, or how to get a stubborn sore to heal; busy surgeons often can't be bothered, answering questions half-heartedly or directing inquiring parents to residents or nurses, who lack training and expertise. Far too often, doctors we encountered were mute when asked to share some of their prized information. In some cases, they were even openly antagonistic, viewing our questions as challenges to their authority.

Early on, when we were debating what to do about Cary's feet, we arranged for a consult with a well-known orthopedic surgeon. Tall, strikingly handsome, and imperious, it was all he could do to look us in the eye, let alone engage in conversation.

The question we were trying to resolve was whether to operate on Cary's clubfeet, or to continue casting them indefinitely. Thus far, we had received diametrically opposed opinions. Rich Davidson had recommended operating, while doctors at the DuPont Institute in Wilmington, Delaware, had suggested casting for as long as eighteen months.

"I'd keep casting him every week," Dr. Sylvan Koch said.

"For how long?" Cathy inquired.

Whatever it takes. I've had kids in casts for a year."

"What about the impact on the child's development?" Cathy asked. "Doesn't wearing casts indefinitely interfere with things like crawling and walking?"

Koch busied himself at a sink. "Look, I don't know what you want to hear," he shouted over the running water. "That's the way I treat bilateral clubfeet. I cast them."

"What's your success rate?" Cathy asked.

"What do you mean?" Koch had turned off the water and turned around. Dissatisfaction clouded his eyes.

"How often do you lose the correction after the casts come off?"

"That's a problem systemic to spina bifida. It doesn't matter whether you're doing surgery or casting. The feet have a tendency to turn back in," Koch said.

"Not according to the medical literature," Cathy boldly replied. She then proceeded to quote chapter and verse the arguments for and against casting. Her tone was polite but firm. Her words, technical and precisely phrased.

Later, we would both remark on how Koch's jaw had dropped while Cathy questioned his facts and figures. More tellingly, he hadn't even attempted to defend himself by revealing his success rate. About all he had managed to sputter before hurrying out the door was a sarcastic remark about Cathy's knowledge of anatomy.

"No way will that man ever touch my child," Cathy said as we stood amid the debris of the broken conversation. To make matters worse, Koch had misplaced the X-rays we had mailed him of Cary's feet, maintaining that he never received them. A week after our visit, his secretary called to report that she had located the pictures. They had been buried under a pile of junk in the doctor's office.

On another occasion, when we were debating what to do about Cary's hips, we arranged a consultation with a prominent surgeon at another medical center in the Philadelphia area.

Noel Wheeler was an imposing curmudgeon, with a shock of white hair, peaked, wizardlike eyebrows, and piercing eyes. Long used to lofty praise from dutiful colleagues and unquestioning residents, Wheeler startled at our innocent questions and allowed for no dissent. As we discovered quickly enough, it was his way or the highway.

On the day of our visit, Wheeler literally exploded into our sad little examining room, tossed a cookie at Cary, and slapped an X-ray of our son's dislocated hips on a wall screen.

"What the hell are we going to do about these?" he boomed at one of the residents who had trailed along on his long white coattails.

While the resident spewed forth information about the

status of Cary's hips, Wheeler tapped a foot impatiently and looked around the room. It was hard to say who was more surprised, Cathy and I, or the gaggle of doctors, nurses, and physical therapists crowded into the tiny cubbyhole.

Wheeler, too, took note of Cathy's impressive medical knowledge (she had briefly studied physiology and had worked for a time as an athletic trainer). "You've been studying up, that's good," he barked. But when Cathy inquired about the value of a different surgical approach to stabilizing Cary's hips than the one favored by Wheeler, the doctor immediately grew defensive.

"Oh, Lindseth," Wheeler said, waving a hand dismissively. "I taught Lindseth everything he knows."

Richard Lindseth was an orthopedic surgeon based in Indiana who had popularized the other procedure. We had heard intriguing things about his approach, which involved fastening the hips in their sockets with the aid of tendons from the child's stomach. However, little in the way of long-term results had been published in the medical literature.

"Look, I've done thousands of these things," Wheeler continued. "I know what works and what doesn't. These other things would take a lot of magic. You don't want to believe me, that's up to you."

Cathy tried to make clear we were seeking guidance, not challenging Wheeler's beliefs. But Wheeler was already halfway out the door.

"Go see Lindseth for all I care," he shouted back at us. Then in a lower, grumbling voice, "Let Lindseth do it."

A moment later Wheeler was gone, never to be heard from again.

Cathy looked from me to the nurses. "What was that all

about?" she asked in a dazed tone. "Did I say something wrong?"

Several of the nurses and therapists shook their heads.

"Is he always like that?" we asked.

"I'll go find out what the story is," one of the nurses said. Soon the room was empty.

I looked at Cary. He was sitting quietly on the examining table. Wheeler hadn't even touched him, let alone examined his hips. "Daddy," Cary said, "I don't think I want this cookie." He handed me the crumbly butter cookie, which I slipped into my coat pocket. "That's okay," I whispered. "I don't think I want this doctor."

Was it us? Were we expecting too much? Were we threatening these doctors somehow? Would we be better off to play the role of supplicant parents?

Cathy and I asked ourselves these questions repeatedly. In the end, we came to trust our own instincts. We had educated ourselves and were painfully aware of the limits of medicine. All we were doing was trying to make the best decisions within those narrow boundaries, trying to do the best we could for Cary.

What so many doctors fail to realize is that they are treating the parents as much as they are their children.

"Children don't make decisions about their care, parents do," Cathy pointed out after one especially frustrating visit. "When are these doctors going to realize that? They blow through the office and throw a few things at you, without any context, and then they blow out again. How do they expect us to make the right choices?"

EIGHT

Clinic

Unlike an acute illness, which is intense but relatively brief, a disabling condition like spina bifida never loosens its ferocious grip on the body. As an infant grows into a toddler, or a teenager into an adult, the issues may change, but they never subside.

This single fact is what distinguishes the care of chronically ill and disabled children from all others. Theirs is a life of constant need and attention, of doctors' visits and hospital stays, of missed opportunities and social isolation stemming from the demands of their imperfect bodies.

According to a 1984 report by Stephen L. Gortmaker and William Sappenfield, "Children with chronic diseases utilize more services and a much wider variety of services than other children."★ They spend four times as many days in the hospital as other children; are seen by physicians twice as frequently; use six times the therapy and support services, require twice as many prescriptions, and also are twice as likely to need braces, wheelchairs, hearing aids, and transportation services.

Our own experience paralleled these academic findings.

During Cary's first year of life, we made approximately fifty trips to hospitals, more than two dozen visits to John Tedeschi's office in Cherry Hill, and another half-dozen visits to outpatient imaging centers for X-rays, CT scans, and MRI procedures. Cary was operated on three times, wore casts for upward of nine months, and was fitted for his first set of braces around the age of one. In addition to these services, Cary attended an Early Intervention Program several days a week, where he was seen by a nurse, physical, occupational, and speech therapists, as well as specialists who charted his social and intellectual progress. When we added it all up, we estimate that Cary received at least one medical service at least every other day that first year.

It did not take a genius to realize that someone had to be responsible for coordinating this mosaic of medical care. The question was who?

The number of candidates was surprisingly limited. Ideally, I suppose, this role would have been filled by one of our pediatricians, or perhaps a nurse or a physician's assistant. Failing that, perhaps our insurer would have appointed one of its many medical directors or nurses to

★"Chronic Childhood Disorders: Prevalence and Impact," *The Pediatric Clinics of North America*, Philadelphia: W. B. Saunders Co., Feb. 1984.

help us through the labyrinthine health-care system. As it turned out, neither of these ideas was especially realistic—reasonable perhaps, but not realistic.

For a variety of reasons, some financial, others having to do with training and practice, physicians haven't been quick to embrace the role of medical ombudsman. Many are simply too busy to spend the time helping parents and patients sift through conflicting medical information. Their practices are small businesses, after all, and depend on volume. Some doctors just don't want to be bothered; they want to make diagnoses and treat patients, not juggle appointments with specialists, critique surgical techniques, and schedule tests and X-rays.

It is also true, however, that insurers provide physicians with few financial incentives to act as ombudsmen. Oh, they talk a good game about paying doctors a premium to serve as case managers. But what they are really talking about is controlling costs, not managing the comprehensive health-care needs of chronically ill children. Few insurers are willing to pay doctors a little extra to make sure these children get all of the care they need.

Paradoxically, were insurers willing to pay pediatricians a little more up front, they would most likely save themselves money in the long run. Potential problems would be identified and treated sooner. Children would get routine preventive care. And instead of fumbling their way from specialist to specialist until they found the right one, parents would be coached on how to choose the right doctor.

Yet, even while they carp about the soaring costs of medical care, insurers continue to follow a course that is penny-wise but pound foolish when dealing with disabled and chronically ill children. Spina bifida is a perfect example.

Instead of recognizing it as a chronic condition with medical consequences lasting a lifetime, insurers act as though each trip to the doctor, hospital, and specialist is an isolated episode. This "à la carte" mentality fosters any number of problems, including a blizzard of paperwork and red tape, duplication of services, inefficiency, and bad medicine. Inevitably, it also increases the cost of care.

Now, assume for a moment that you are the insurer. Wouldn't it make sense to identify all of your subscribers with spina bifida and other disabling conditions, find out what services they need, and then negotiate arrangements with hospitals and doctors to provide that care?

Countless studies have shown that if you can identify a problem early enough you can treat it successfully and save money at the same time. Similarly, if you can develop a select network of providers who concentrate on caring for disabled and chronically ill children, they will gain experience and be better at their work. That should benefit the patients and pocketbooks of the insurers.

If it makes so much sense, then how come insurers are reluctant to do it?

The short answer is: Why bother? If you're already making a profit, where's the incentive to change? Recall that insurers essentially operate like banks. They collect our premiums in advance and invest the money. Claims filter in and checks are mailed out. Only HMOs make any pretense at managing care, and even here, they are generally referring to managing the cost of care, not the care itself.

The longer, more involved answer has to do with the nature of medical insurance and the industry's idea of what constitutes risk. Health insurance was created to protect individuals against the ruinous consequences of a catastrophic illness, for example a heart attack, brain tumor, or car accident, requiring a lengthy hospital stay. It was never intended to pay for chronic conditions such as spina bifida or cerebral palsy, which are incapacitating but not necessarily life-threatening.

As far as insurers are concerned, there is no risk in chronic illness. Disabled children fall outside the margins of medical underwriting, if not explicitly, then certainly implicitly. This results in any number of absurd situations.

For instance, an insurer will pay for a bone marrow transplant, open heart surgery, or experimental cancer treatment costing upward of one hundred thousand dollars, but refuse to pay for a physical therapist to manipulate a child's muscles once a week at a cost of $30. The rationale: one is life-threatening, unpredictable, and treated in a hospital. The other isn't life-threatening, is part of a pattern of care, thus predictable, and the care takes place in the home or an office setting.

Paradoxically, if a disabled child requires surgery because his knees or hips have locked with contractures, something that can be prevented through physical therapy, the insurer will fork over $5,000 or $10,000 for the procedure. Similarly, insurers will refuse to pay for a wheelchair for a child with cerebral palsy, but cover the expense of surgery, casting, and therapy if the same child stumbles and breaks a leg. Go figure.

It wasn't supposed to be this way.

During the seventies, a movement took hold to create specialty clinics, usually based in teaching hospitals, for children with disabling conditions. There, the theory went, they could be followed by teams of specialists in a coordinated fashion.

For example, at a spina bifida clinic, a neurosurgeon would be responsible for the brain. A urologist would be responsible for the kidneys, bladder, and bowel. An orthopedic surgeon would watch over the spine, hips, knees, and feet. A physical therapist would survey the child's muscles and tendons. A developmental pediatrician would follow the child's medical, intellectual, and social progress. And a social worker would tend to the child's and family's emotional needs.

It was a wonderful idea. Instead of running from doctor to doctor, children could be treated under one roof. Families could establish lasting relationships with physicians. Ideas could be exchanged, new therapies explored. All for the low cost of about $300 per visit.

Unfortunately, clinics work a lot better on paper than they do in practice.

It has been our experience while visiting four different clinics in the Philadelphia area that they are organized first and foremost for the convenience of doctors and the training of unseasoned medical residents, not for the care of children.

The clinics tend to be oversubscribed, marked by long waiting periods and then short bursts of activity when a doctor appears. Most are staffed by residents only a year or two out of medical school. While perfectly competent in routine matters, they possess little if any expertise in the specific illness or condition. In fact, they often know less than the parents, which, when you think about it, makes sense. By definition a resident is an inexperienced doctor. He or she is in clinic to learn, not to lead or counsel parents in the subtleties of surgical procedures and cutting-edge therapies.

I recall one time in particular when Cathy asked one of the urology residents at St. Christopher's a question about Cary's bladder, which we were told was undersized and had an open neck, resulting in dribbling.★ The poor fellow didn't have a clue what she was asking him and ended up repeating the same answer like a broken record. Cathy finally asked him how long he had been attached to the clinic. "To be honest, I've only been in the clinic about a month," he responded. I had to step out of the examining room to keep from laughing.

If we were lucky, an attending physician accompanied the resident as backup, filling in the gaps. But they were often so busy all they did was pop in long enough to say hello and pop back out again. At one clinic, the attendings frequently didn't even show up. We went one eighteen-month stretch without seeing a urologist or neurosurgeon because they were either in surgery or traveling to conferences.

"I don't know what I would do if, God forbid, Cary's shunt failed or he had a problem with his kidneys," Cathy said following one clinic. "How are we supposed to have any confidence in these people if we never see them?"

Needless to say, we were left to manage all of Cary's medical needs.

When Cary was two months old we took him to his first clinic for a checkup. We were shocked when one of the

★Shortly after Cary turned six, another urologist and his nurse-assistant tested Cary and concluded that his bladder wasn't nearly so small, and didn't have an open neck. Instead of having to undergo surgery, he may be able to empty his bladder by using a catheter every three or four hours.

doctors warned us to look away. He was going to insert a catheter into Cary's penis and up into his bladder to drain urine. "You can watch if you want, but sometimes parents feel a little squeamish at first," he explained.

That's odd, I thought. Why doesn't he just put a bag on Cary if he wants a urine sample?

The answer came to me later. He wasn't collecting a sample. He was demonstrating how to catheterize a boy for the female resident who had been observing the session.

The more I thought about it, the angrier I became. The doctor hadn't bothered to ask our permission, let alone explain why he was performing the procedure. He had sprung it on us with only the most perfunctory of warnings. More important, he hadn't even chosen a good subject. Cary had a tiny, dysfunctional bladder that failed to hold urine. Inserting a catheter was futile; there wasn't sufficient fluid to drain. Had the doctor bothered to examine Cary's bladder, he would have known this. He was too busy teaching. Or else he didn't care.

Shortly thereafter, we began to take Cary to the spina bifida clinic at St. Christopher's Hospital for Children, a teaching facility affiliated with Temple University. Old and broken, St. Christopher's was a poor stepchild to the newer and wealthier Children's Hospital. Its neglected campus in North Philadelphia frightened many first-time visitors unaccustomed to the sight of bombed-out row houses, graffiti-scrawled buildings, and open, littered lots. Cramped, chaotic, and undersized, it also suffered from a bit of an inferiority complex, although the level of medicine practiced there was first rate.

What St. Christopher's lacked in amenities and financial resources, it more than made up for in spirit. The clinic staff was friendly, hardworking, and competent. The nurses and doctors went out of their way to make parents feel welcome. Questions were encouraged and expected. It didn't matter how many you had or how long it took to answer them. Here, the staff actually paused to chat and trade stories. It was a revelation and a breath of fresh air.

The acting director, Julia Hayes, was a sturdy yet mild-mannered pediatrician, with dark locks of hair and a quick wit. She was thorough, encouraging without seeming patronizing, and playful with the baby, no small gift in a doctor. At one point, she lifted Cary over her head, holding him face down, to see if he tightened his neck muscles. "He's a little floppy," she said, referring to his muscle tone, "but not enough to worry about. It's just something he needs to work on."

Ray Truex, a skilled neurosurgeon, was a quiet, funny little man with exquisite hands. As is any acclaimed medical man, he was trailed by an entourage of residents everywhere he went. When they crowded into our tiny cubicle, it was like the long, luminous tail of a comet crashing through the atmosphere.

A fastidious dresser, who favored expensive tweed jackets, Truex was wearing a cranberry tie with hunting dogs the day we first met. Bending over to examine our naked four-month-old son, he suddenly caught himself and tucked his tie inside his shirt. "I've lost a lot of good ties doing this," he said.

The reference flew by Cathy.

Truex smiled. Then, meekly pointing in the direction of Cary's penis, he made a small hissing sound.

"Oh, I get it," Cathy chuckled. "I bet you have."

For all of his brilliance, Truex was quick to compliment the work of Leslie Sutton. "He's done a fine job," he said, examining Cary's back and shunt. "You should be pleased."

The person responsible for making sure that the clinic ran smoothly was Ricki Hobdell, the head nurse. Medium-built, with cropped, sandy hair and a shy smile, Ricki was at once anchor, negotiator, politician, schedule master, and counselor. She played all of these roles with equal skill and was well liked by parents. If there was a question that needed answering, Ricki took care of it. A referral required, you should see Ricki. A shoulder to cry on, Ricki could be counted on. Without Ricki, the clinic surely would have collapsed into chaos.

As it was, it began to unravel of its own accord.

First, Julia Hayes resigned. That had been expected. But it was still a blow. Then Ray Truex left without warning or explanation in the beginning of our second year in clinic. One day we showed up for clinic and he was gone. When we asked why, the doctors and nurses were tight-lipped. Even the new director, David Schor, said he didn't know. "Apparently it's something personal," he said.

During the next four years, the clinic continued to be plagued by turnover. Truex's replacement, Jogi Patisipu, whom we also admired, lasted about eighteen months. We discovered he had been gone for several months when we arrived for another visit. Again, there had been no warning or notification.

With Patisipu gone, I expressed concern about the absence of a neurosurgeon in clinic. What if Cary's shunt had failed during this period? Who would we have contacted? Who would have done the surgery?

Schor deflected my questions. Another neurosurgeon had already been hired, he explained, and would be in place by our next visit. Later, I learned from sources at

Temple that Patisipu had been the victim of infighting within the different surgeons' camps. Disgusted, he had moved on to another hospital in Florida.

Turnovers also plagued the supporting services. In five years, the clinic had five physical therapists and at least four different social workers. It got so that we didn't know who Cary's doctors were supposed to be, let alone had any confidence in what they said.

Early in the summer of 1991, I called Schor to complain. I did so reluctantly because I liked the modest director and thought he was trying his best to hold the place together. But forces beyond his control were dragging the clinic down. In addition to the turnover problem, attending physicians weren't showing up, leaving parents to earnest but inexperienced residents. Morale had also soured. It was as though the staff realized that clinic was a low-budget, low-priority event in a high-tech setting and had started to behave that way.

"I don't understand," I began my conversation with Schor. "What is the point of holding a clinic if the attendings don't bother to show up, or if they only show up for a few minutes? During our recent visit, you were the only attending we saw. What good does that do the parents and children?"

"I agree with you it's not the best if the attendings aren't appearing," Schor conceded. "That's something I am aware of and think we can do a better job at."

However, Schor then tried to lay the problem at the feet of the residents. "If there're questions they can't handle, they ought to be presenting them to the attendings. Even if that means getting back to the parents later on to answer their questions."

Schor was missing the point as far as I was concerned.

The idea was to have the attendings at the clinic, not play phone tag whenever we had a question. "Who is going to follow up?" I demanded to know. "In five years, I think we have received one follow-up phone call and that wasn't a doctor. The purpose of the clinic ought to be providing the best possible care to these children, not serving as a proving ground for residents, which right now is all it is."

Agitated, I unloaded all of the anger and frustration that had been building up inside of me for years.

"If medicine can retrieve the heart of a dead man, pack it in ice, fly it hundreds or even thousands of miles to another hospital, where a team of specially trained doctors and nurses transplant it into the chest of another dying person and kick start it to life, is it too much to ask a few doctors to gather once a month to examine these children and offer their parents some help?"

"I agree with you that clinical care is the first reason this or any other hospital exists," Schor said. "But the reality is that this hospital also serves an important role as a medical training institution. It's my personal belief that these two roles don't have to be mutually exclusive. At least that is what we are striving for."

"Do you think you are balancing those roles now?"

Schor paused. "Probably not as well as we should be. I don't think you would be calling if we were."

"I wouldn't be calling if there wasn't a problem," I said.

Schor said he would pass along our concerns to the clinic staff. "Anonymously, of course."

Three days later, a form letter arrived from Schor announcing several staff changes at the clinic and the creation of a family support program. "I have asked each staff member to be sure to listen to your questions and concerns at each visit," Schor wrote. "I would like to suggest that you write down any such items before clinic and give them to Ricki when you sign in."

"Funny, but isn't that the way they do it at research conventions?" I asked Cathy.

"Read on," she said. "It goes downhill from there."

I scanned the page. Buried at the bottom was an announcement from Schor that he was leaving St. Christopher's, effective at the end of the month, to take a job out of state.★

"I don't believe it. I spend all of this time complaining about staff turnover, and he didn't have the decency to say he was leaving? This is incredibly depressing."

"I know."

It got worse. Shortly thereafter, the clinic conducted a survey to find out what were the most important medical needs of the 150 children it followed. The overwhelming response was bowel management. Because most children with spina bifida are unable to control their bowels, they have to use high-fiber diets, enemas, suppositories, and biofeedback to empty themselves. It is a daily struggle, and probably the single most frustrating, humiliating, and exhausting task encountered by these children and their parents.

Given the significance of the problem, one might think that the clinic and hospital would develop a program to help the children and investigate new aids. But neither did. "Unfortunately, our . . . clinic does not have a formal

---

★Schor was replaced by Maureen Fee. The third director in five years, Fee was direct, competent, and sensitive to parents' needs. But as of this writing, it was too soon to tell whether she could stabilize the clinic.

Bowel Maintenance Program. This matter is being investigated and any information will be shared in a future newsletter," parents were informed in a July 1991 letter.

We were growing convinced that the clinic and these children were not an especially high priority of the hospital.

About the same time, St. Christopher's opened a new $100 million hospital with a spacious center court, atrium, garden eating area, and towering parking deck. We had high hopes that the new building in a less-gritty location would help to revitalize the clinic.

When we visited the new facility for our clinic, however, we were sorely disappointed. The guards at the information desk didn't know where it was being held, nor did they seem to know how to find out.

"Maybe it's listed in the hospital directory," I suggested.

No such luck. Nor were there any signs. Finally, after bouncing in and out of several departments, I found the clinic tucked away on the backside of a third-floor hallway in a tiny, unadorned room, now overflowing with parents and children.

Once more, the message seemed to be that children with spina bifida should be neither seen, nor heard.

What should we do?

Cathy and I went back and forth. In the summer of 1991 we concluded if medicine wasn't going to work with us, we would have to make it work for us. We would have to put together our own network of specialists and look at abandoning the clinic. We were weary of making excuses for doctors, second-guessing ourselves, and wondering if we were doing everything we could for Cary. It was time to expend our energy on more positive things.

NINE

Under the Deforming Heel

The five-year-old girl with the broken leg was what was known as a "screamer" around the cluttered, highly informal casting room at Children's Hospital.

Even before Joe, the droll, dark-haired technician from South Philly, had turned on his saw, she had broken into deep sobs and had begun clinging to her mother.

"It's okay, it's okay," her mother repeated, stroking her daughter's neck. "They're just going to cut the cast off. Don't you want your regular leg back?"

The little girl was not impressed, and when Joe switched on the high-pitched saw, her sobs turned to ear-piercing wails.

Cary, who was in for new casts on his feet and was propped on a nearby table, stared serenely at the ruckus.

"Well, at least somebody's taking this well," Rich Davidson, Cary's orthopedic surgeon, said as he passed by. "It will only be a minute or two."

Actually, it was more like ten or fifteen minutes. Each time Joe tried to maneuver the saw toward the cast, the girl lurched away. Finally, a couple of residents who had been hanging around moved in and held her legs.

The poor girl howled so she didn't notice at first that Joe had sliced the cast neatly in two and was holding it for her to see. When it finally registered, her sobs turned into big, broken laughs. "Hey," she cried, in a surprised tone, "that didn't hurt. I feel better. Hey, I feel better. Mom, look, my cast is off."

Joe folded the cast together and handed it to the girl. "You might like to have this as a souvenir," he said. The little girl happily accepted the gift.

It took a sense of humor to work in the casting room. One encountered horrible deformities day after day caused by rioting genes, withered joints, and bones splintered by a mind-boggling assortment of accidents. As if that weren't bad enough, it was the job of the technicians and orthopedic surgeons who labored here to immobilize the legs and arms and feet—indeed, sometimes the entire bodies—of normally active children. In many cases, that meant the children no longer could run or jump or play.

Joe and the other technicians dealt with the dark side of their work by poking fun at what they did. An entire wall was lined with outlandishly decorated leg casts saved over the years and served as a veritable walking tour of the mood of the nation. There were flower casts and psychedelic casts and intricately patterned casts and angry, power-to-the-people casts. There were casts autographed in English and casts autographed in Spanish. There was even a cast or two autographed in an Asian-language dialect, donated by a group in West Philadelphia.

Someone had placed a neon-yellow rubber chicken above one counter that had been encased in a full-body cast. A sign read: CHICKEN BODY CAST AWARD.

Even the doctors seemed different down here—more relaxed, able to laugh at themselves, confident in an athlete's pumped-up way but also not afraid to admit defeat. If the operating room was their workshop, the clinic was where they saw the results of their work, often for the first time. It was a humbling, busy, awesome place, more akin to a garage shop than a hospital clinic, littered with tools, gauze, past, casts, and dust. It was okay to roll up one's sleeves here and get a little dirty while you tinkered and hammered and cut. That was expected, the nature of the work. If neurologists were the engineers of the medical profession, charting the nervous highways of the body, and plastic surgeons were the landscape artists, trimming noses and inflating breasts, then orthopods were the drywall builders and plasterers, ripping out damaged bones and tendons, manipulating or replacing them and encasing them again in a canopy of gauze and paste.

It was here, against a booming background of rock music, that Rich Davidson first pulled out a skeleton of the foot to illustrate how Cary's feet had twisted at sharp right angles during gestation. Simply put, our son's heel bones had not dropped as far down as they should have, resulting in a crowded arrangement of bones that had forced his feet to roll inward. Davidson would correct the defect by releasing several tendons that held Cary's feet, and "drop his heels" so his feet flattened to a weight-bearing position. Stainless-steel pins would hold the correction. But it would still be necessary to cast Cary's feet every week or so.

The surgery took place in September 1986, when Cary was nearly five months old. I took off from work to escort him to the hospital, where he and I arrived groggy-eyed and hungry, at around 7:00 A.M. Even at that ungodly hour, the Short Procedure Unit was backed out into the hallway with edgy parents and children. Poor Cary hadn't been allowed to eat after midnight and was starving. I gave him a pacifier and did everything possible to keep him entertained as our scheduled time for surgery came and went. Luckily, Cary seemed to sense that something special was taking place, and couldn't have been more cooperative. When I finally handed him over to a nurse around noon, I had tears in my eyes.

About two hours later, Davidson appeared in the waiting area in his green surgical garb. "Everything went well. There were no hitches, no problems at all," he said, kneading his hands.

Two months later, during a follow-up visit, he asked permission to show Cary's feet to the mother of an infant girl with clubfeet. "See how nice and straight they look after surgery." The mother looked pleased. Davidson even took a picture for his records, and we kidded him about receiving royalties.

But before a year, we noticed that Cary's feet were begining to turn inward again. When we mentioned this to Davidson, he was doubtful at first and told us we had to expect some loss of correction. But the problem got worse, month by month, until finally, Cary's feet were twisted so badly they wouldn't fit into the plastic molds he wore while sleeping.

Davidson operated again in March of 1989, releasing additional tendons and this time the correction held. By this point, Cary was an old hand at hospitals. When the nurses rolled him out of the recovery area, he was already awake and singing to himself. Later, when I visited after work, I found him sitting up in his bed, listening to a Raffi tape on Cathy's headphones and sipping a vanilla milk-shake.

Little by little, Cary showed us the way.

His progress wasn't always neat and symmetrical, as in a textbook, and Cathy and I spent a good deal of time fretting over schedules and timetables, but in his own singular style, Cary managed to pile up his share of victories during these challenging first years.

Most would be considered fairly routine milestones in the life of a normal infant or toddler. Tasks like sitting, crawling, and walking are thrilling but expected accomplishments for these children. However, for Cary, who faced daunting physical obstacles, no milestone was routine. Each presented a special set of challenges, knots, and puzzles, and was all the more special as a result.

Cary got lots of help along the way, especially from Cathy and Sue Cheney, a dedicated physical therapist in his early-intervention program. Still, it was up to him to master each task, and as with any young child, he occasionally objected. Only when Cary said *no* he meant it. No amount of pleas, reasoning, or bribes would win him over. As we would discover soon enough, the phrase "single-minded" was coined with Cary Gaul in mind. Fortunately, this same spirit and determination were also our allies, and helped him overcome countless hurdles, starting virtually from the day he was born.

One of the earliest concerns we had was over Cary's ability to control his head. Julia Hayes had noted during our clinic visit that Cary had "marked head lag and hypotonia," or low muscle tone in his neck. As a result, his head tended to flop from side to side like a Raggedy Andy doll when placed in a sitting position.

To strengthen Cary's neck muscles, we placed a rolled-up towel under his chest for support while he was lying down. This made it a little easier to push his head up and hold it stationary. In no time at all, he was supporting himself for thirty seconds while he looked around the room for familiar faces and toys.

When Julia Hayes tested Cary again in the fall of 1986, he was like a different baby, tucking his head against his chest when she held him upside down and performing like a star during games she used to test his fine motor skills.

"Developmentally he [Cary] is doing fine," Hayes noted in a follow-up report. "He knows his parents and is not yet afraid of strangers. He has said "mom-mom." He imitates sounds, reaches for objects, and he has a raking grab. He releases objects. He can roll from his abdomen to his back. Occasionally he blows raspberries and makes a very strange noise, but this noise occurs only when he is playing. It never occurs when he is angry, upset, crying, or asleep."

After weeks and weeks of practice, Cary learned to sit all by himself about the age of ten months. It occurred during a break in one of his physical therapy sessions at the early-intervention program. Cathy and Sue Cheney were chatting when Cathy suddenly looked up to find Cary sitting on a mat examining some neon-colored plastic rings. "Hey, look," she shouted. "Cary's sitting!"

"Hey, you're right," Sue cried.

In normal situations, children learn to sit at around six months. It had taken Cary nearly twice as long because he lacked control over his upper body. Even when propped by pillows, he tumbled forward like a bowling pin.

Cathy wiped a tear from her eye. "I can't believe it," she said, taking in her son. "I was beginning to think he'd never do it."

Sue broke into a big smile. Athletically built, with curly brown hair down to her shoulders, Sue had rapidly become a friend and counselor at a time when we were groping for direction. "Way to go Cary," she exclaimed.

Cary dropped the toy he was playing with and looked at Sue and Cathy. He didn't know what the fuss was about, but smiled anyway, breaking into a long, slow belly laugh until he finally lost his balance and crashed.

As Cary became more proficient at sitting, he took to rocking furiously back and forth whenever he became excited. We first noticed this unusual behavior when he was about eleven months old. One day, our two cats happened to wander by him. Cary desperately wanted at them. Unable to crawl or talk, his way of showing he was excited was to rock. Later on, the rocking became generalized, a way of entertaining himself and having some fun. Just about anything might set him off: the cats, a voice, the TV or radio, his brother racing through the house. We were certain he was going to tip over and split his skull. We could just see the scene in the emergency room.

"Exactly how did this happen, Mr. and Mrs. Gaul?"

"He tipped over, Doctor, while he was rocking like a madman."

"Excuse me. Could you repeat that? I thought you said he tipped over?"

We wondered: Could parents be arrested for child neglect for allowing their kid to tip over?

Fortunately, for us, Cary never crashed, and eventually outgrew the rocking.

Cary continued to wear casts while his feet healed, and the combination of that extra weight and missing muscles and nerves in his legs prevented him from exploring all but his immediate world.

We worried about this lack of motion, and with good reason. Movement is probably the single most important factor in an infant's development. It is the foundation for walking, exploring, cognitive development, and, ultimately, independence and a sense of self-mastery. If an infant is not free to investigate and manipulate the world around him, it may stunt his development and impinge on his sense of competency. Some researchers contend that the high rate of visual-perceptual problems in children with spina bifida stems from the fact that while infants, they do not see and move through the environment the same way as other children.

As much as we could, we brought the world to Cary. Toys, tapes, books, games. Still, it was not the same because he was depending on us, not moving out on his own.

At eight months, Cary figured out how to push himself up into a crouch and roll back and forth on his knees. But when he tried to move forward, he ended up sliding backward or turning helplessly in a circle. Because he had no control over his feet, he couldn't use them to thrust himself ahead. Without sensation in his knees, he also couldn't tell where the lower third of his body was at any given time, which made reciprocal crawling all but impossible.

The first breakthrough came when Cary's casts came off in December 1986. Freed from those heavy shackles, he was suddenly able to roll anywhere he wanted and maneuver into a scooting position without any trouble. From there, he started to rock back and forth on his arms and eye his toys. Finally, four days before his first birthday, he discovered that if he thrust ahead from his rocking position he could propel himself forward, like an inchworm. It wasn't crawling in any classic sense, but who cared? It worked. Cary could get to his toys, and we were encouraged that our son was making progress.

Over the months, Cary refined his crawling technique so that he was scooting around our house chasing the cats, following his big brother and parents, and generally getting into anything that wasn't placed out of his reach.

By the time he was fifteen months old, Cary was crawling on his knees, one leg after another, or scooting on his buttocks, like a crab. His ability to explore exploded. One minute he was on our front porch playing with his toys, the next he was in the kitchen checking out the cabinets or on his way up the steps to a landing where we had a large poster of a gray cat. One day when Cathy was in the kitchen, she heard a *thump thump thump* and came running. She found Cary at the bottom of the steps. At first, she thought he had taken a tumble. But he was grinning from ear to ear and singing a little song: *de de de de*. She watched him crawl back up the steps, flop onto his tummy, and come sliding down. "You little devil," she cried. That evening at supper she recalled the entire episode. "He scared me half to death," she said.

We also had a big backyard, with flower beds and a

sandbox, which Cary enjoyed exploring. About the only thing he couldn't do was keep up with the other kids. Our neighborhood was full of boys and they were constantly on the go. But we took solace in the fact that at least he could be near them some of the time. That alone was a major improvement. When he learned to walk, we reasoned, he would be able to take part in their games and blend into the background.

Little could we know how exhilarating and frustrating walking would prove to be.

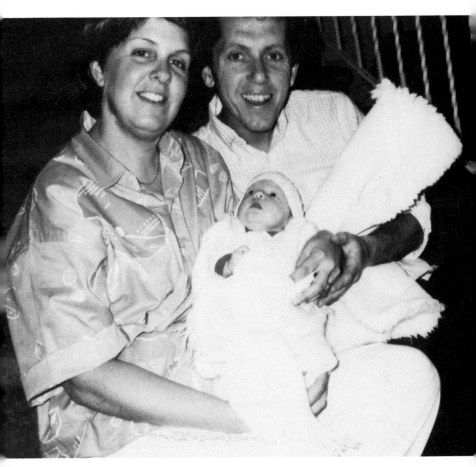

Cary was all eyes for his mom the evening we brought him home.

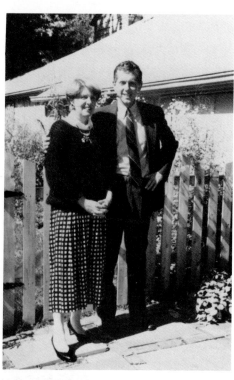

Cathy and I at the new house before heading to New York.

With therapist Sue Chaney at the early-intervention program.

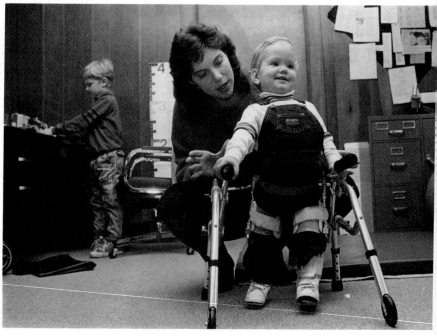

Cary with his first pair of braces.

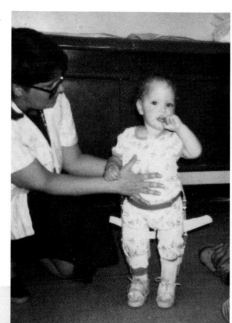

Cary and I at the Jersey Shore.

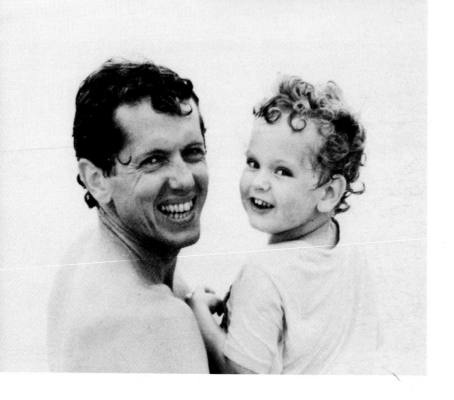

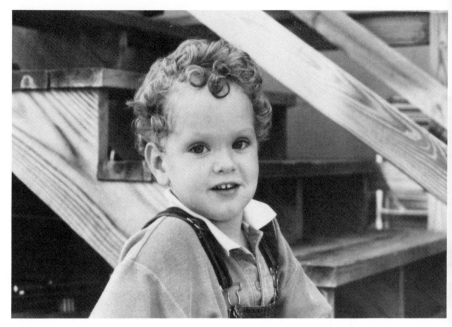

Cary at age five.

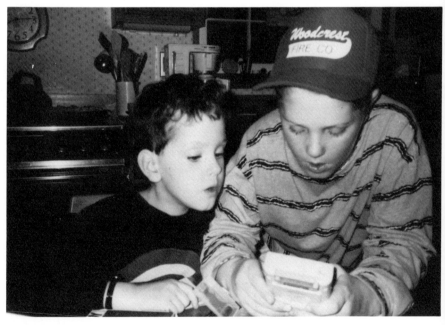

Greg and Cary playing a video game on Cary's sixth birthday.

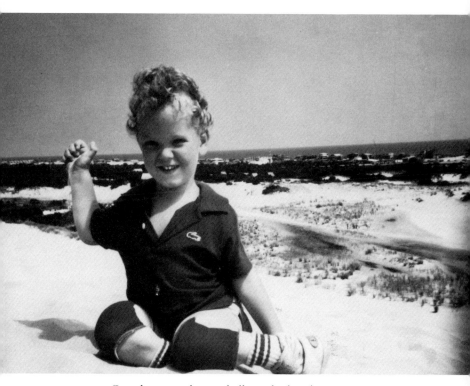

Cary loves to throw shells at the beach.

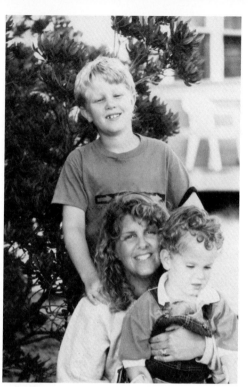

Cathy and the boys at the Jersey Shore.

Cathy and Cary on the beach.

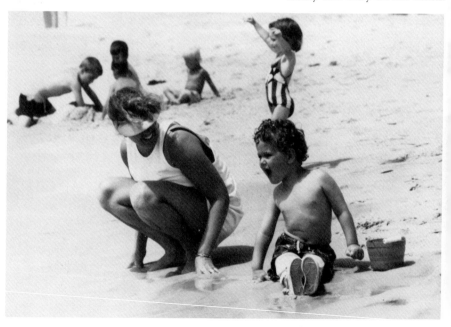

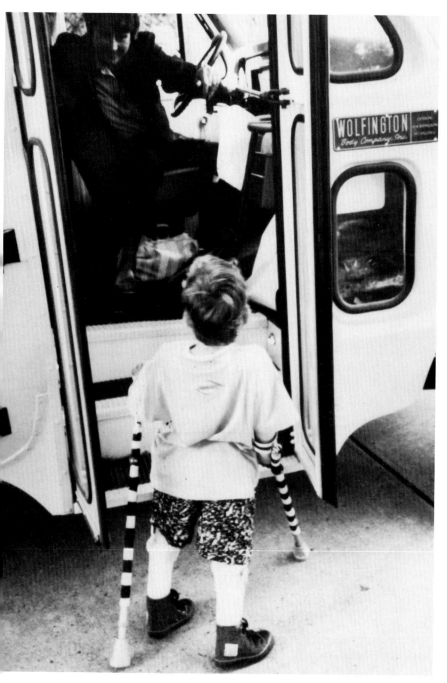

Greeting his bus driver before kindergarten.

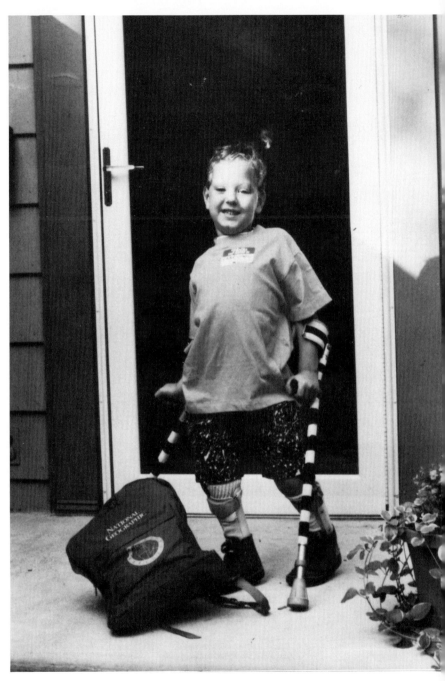

The first day of school.

TEN

Confucius Says

Our greatest glory is not in never falling but in rising every time we fall.

—CONFUCIUS

At the age of fourteen months, Cary received his first set of braces, and his and our lives became of whirlwind of emotion.

Overnight he found himself caged from his hips to his toes in a scaffolding of stainless steel, leather, plastic, and velcro. Not surprisingly, he didn't want to have anything to do with them, protesting every time we tried to put them on and even crying at the mere sight of them. Having experienced the freedom of crawling, all he wanted was to be left alone to explore. It was too much for any child his age to understand.

His tears worked on us, slicing through our defenses and leaving us raw and weak. Wavering, we allowed our doubts the upper hand. We started to look for excuses to skip a day, only to awaken the following morning feeling guilty. Clearly, this was something that was going to take time to understand and come to terms with.

Paradoxically, a part of me thought that once Cary got his braces he would be up and walking. Why not? Each day, thousands of toddlers across America take their first wobbly steps toward independence. Cary was late. But now he had the means to join the parade.

I don't know what I was thinking. I suppose, with hindsight, I wasn't really thinking at all. I was dreaming. Wishing my way to a more charitable future I had carved out in a corner of my brain.

How was I to know it would take months, even years, to perfect this seemingly simple undertaking. With Cary, we not only were starting from scratch, we were also reinventing the process, angle by angle, joint by joint, muscle by muscle, one excruciating step at a time, until we were finally in a position to begin the real work.

We began modestly enough by trying to get Cary to accept wearing his braces for brief periods of time, slowly increasing these sessions over weeks and months until they lasted for an hour or two. In the beginning, big crocodile tears rolled down his face, and we had to look away or leave the room. Little was accomplished. But just when it seemed like he would never consent, the tears stopped and we began to make progress.

Before Cary could walk, he had to strengthen the muscles in his arms and shoulders so that he could support his weight in a standing position. To do this, Sue Cheney used a kid-sized set of parallel bars and had Cary practice walking from one end to the other. Using the bars for support, he could get used to the idea of lifting and pulling himself forward, the motion he would need later when he started to use a walker.

But how do you entice a stubborn sixteen-month-old toddler into doing something that isn't much fun?

Sue's answer was to place one of Cary's favorite toys on a table at each end of the parallel bars. The idea was simple and effective. Each time Cary negotiated the fifteen feet or so, he was rewarded by being allowed to play for a few minutes. Then he had to turn around and walk back the other way.

We used any number of games, gimmicks, and tricks to motivate Cary during these first difficult months in braces. Most were unadorned and direct. For example, a song or toy or snack. As he grew and the tasks became harder, the rewards also became slightly more elaborate. It was amazing how hard a little boy would work when promised a "Happy Meal" at McDonald's, milk shake, or small toy. Call it bribery or positive reinforcement. Whatever, it worked.

Little by little, Cary made progress. After strengthening his upper body, Sue moved him into a walker with wheels attached to the front legs. The idea was to get him used to the motion of walking but with the walker doing the bulk of the work. Each time Cary inched ahead, the lightweight aluminum safety net rolled with him. As long as he didn't let go, he didn't have to worry about falling. He could go as fast or slow as he wanted. And if something blocked his path, the walker was light enough that he could lift it and maneuver his way around the object.

Once more, Cary balked. The newness of standing frightened him. And he found pushing and controlling the walker at the same time difficult. "I don't blame him for fussing," Cathy said one evening. "No matter what you say, it's still work to him. Why should he have to do all this while the other kids are outside playing?"

A few months into the project, Sue tried unfastening the upper set of locks on Cary's braces, allowing his hips to bend more easily. This seemed to make a big difference. Instead of having to struggle mightily to lift and tug the walker, he could pick up his feet more easily now and the walker would roll along with him.

In January, when it was too cold or snowy for Cary to practice outside, Cathy started going to a nearby mall early in the morning before the stores opened. The smooth surfaces there were ideal for the walker and, at that hour, the only other traffic were the retirees who used the mall for exercise. After a while, Cary and Cathy were regulars. The elderly walkers all recognized them and waved, and the guard even gave them a special pass in case anyone questioned what they were doing.

Up and down the hallways they went, sometimes for an hour or more. Cary looked forward to these trips, which were a veritable paradise of sensory stimulation for a curious toddler. He also enjoyed spying in the store windows, especially of Radio Shack, which displayed the telephones he liked so much. Shrewdly, Cathy positioned Cary across from the store so he had to cross the mall to get there. This simple yet effective incentive worked like a charm. Cary tugged and shuffled his way across the tiles. Some days, if they were running late, the store would be open and Cary got to go inside and play with the phones, with the manager's blessing, of course. Cary became a favorite of the workers. They looked for him and all came by to say hello when he appeared. Cathy and Cary finished their sessions by stopping off at a mall shop that made fresh cinnamon buns. Cary didn't care much for the bun, but how he loved the rich, creamy icing on top, licking it clean every time. Somewhere along the way, he took to calling these treats "cinnamon bunnies," which amused us all no end.

One of my favorite pictures of Cary is of him standing proudly in his walker outside of this shop. He is wearing blue corduroy pants and a bright red sweater with a dinosaur splashed across his chest. His smile explodes across his then-chunky face, lighting his wide blue eyes and the fitful blond curls that tumble and soar on top of his broad forehead. Here is a happy child, pleased with himself and the world, at least for a time, free of any and all shackles.

A few weeks before his second birthday, Sue decided to try Cary in arm crutches that clamped at his elbows. He hated the thin, rubber-tipped poles, and let us all know it, brandishing them above his head like swords and screaming bloody murder whenever Sue came near.

"He'll cooperate when he's good and ready," Cathy observed one evening during this rather extended siege. "I know the way he operates. He'll fight it and fight it until he realizes what it can do for him. Then one day it will be done."

I was encouraged to see Cathy had a smile on her face. It helped to have a sense of humor at times like this.

Weeks passed. Cary turned two and we could hardly believe it. Cathy planned a large family gathering to celebrate both of the boys' birthdays (Greg had turned seven in March), but we had to cancel it at the last minute when everyone except Cary came down with the flu. We settled for a small party at home with a store-bought cake and presents wrapped in tissue paper. Not that it mattered. Cary was thrilled just to blow out his candles and open his presents. His favorites were a toy plane that Disney characters could sit in and several Raffi tapes, which he (and everyone else) listened to constantly. Even today, years later, I still catch myself humming the song "Baby Beluga" for no apparent reason.

Spring arrived that year on the backside of an "onion snow," so named because it comes even as the floppy stalks of onion grass are working their way up through the mottled earth.

One afternoon in late April my telephone rang at work and Cathy was on the other end excitedly explaining how Cary had walked on his own during a physical therapy session at the Kingsway Learning Center.

"He did it! He did it!" she cried. "He actually walked! Oh, Gil, you should have seen it. Everybody was so proud. There wasn't a dry eye in the house."

Sue had positioned herself behind Cary, gripping his elbows for support. Each time she moved one of his arms, he had taken a tiny step forward. One after another, until finally, he had inched ahead on his own.

"His posture wasn't terrific," Cathy said. "But Sue didn't seem to care. She said he'd straighten up when he wasn't so afraid of falling."

It was all I could do to concentrate the rest of the afternoon. Cary had walked! Our little boy had opened the door to freedom. Now all he had to do was slip through it.

Cary practiced through the summer and into the fall. Some days he was a model student who worked diligently at his exercises. At other times he fought Sue and Cathy at every turn.

"Cary not walk today," he would screech, scrunching up his face in a fiery ball of protest. "Go away!"

No one day or episode comes to mind when Cary stopped fighting and decided he wanted to walk. The desire seemed to click in slowly as he realized that there were certain advantages to being on one's feet. Instead of looking up at other kids from ground level, he could now meet them eye to eye. It also was an advantage when reaching for toys and books, or when helping oneself to treats from the refrigerator and pantry.

Around Christmas, Cathy took Cary back to the mall, this time with his crutches. The magical displays and splashy colors enticed Cary from one store to another. He also enjoyed walking to a fountain located at one of the far ends of the mall. There, to the delight of the oldsters, he happily pitched penny after penny into the foaming water.

Cary gradually became an accomplished walker. With increased mobility came a new boldness and a heightened desire to explore. The tempo of his journeys around the block increased to a reckless trot. He was also oblivious to bumps and cracks in the sidewalk, thrusting himself up and over on the handgrips of his crutches.

"Cary, you're going to fall," we warned. But, of course, he didn't listen. What three-year-old does?

Every so often he crashed in a frightening heap and we

hurried to pick him up. Most of the time he was more embarrassed than hurt, and we left him to his own devices. Kids in braces are not brittle little stalks that snap upon impact. Quite the contrary. They are just like other kids, taking hundreds of seemingly disastrous spills from which they rise remarkably intact.

Not that it doesn't take some getting used to. The shock of seeing your son topple on a patch of ice or a slippery tile floor, legs and arms crashing at horrific angles, always takes your breath away. Then there is the commotion caused by well-intentioned strangers who, assuming the worst, rush forward to help. How do you explain that falling is part of your son's everyday experience, neither important nor unimportant, until singled out? And that the glory is in rising each time he falls, not in never falling?

Cary accompanied Cathy on nearly all of her errands. Only now, instead of riding in a stroller or cart, he walked. Besides the mall, his favorite places to go were clothing stores, where he played hide and seek among the dusty racks of pants and dresses; food shopping, because Cathy allowed him to roam up and down the aisles, and just about any store that had a telephone and an employee kind enough to let him play with it.

In the winter of 1988, we began to attend a Quaker Meeting near our house. During the hour-long Meeting for Worship, Cary stayed in a day-care program. But afterward we permitted him to wander in the hoary old hall while we chatted with other members. Cary was in heaven, squeezing down the narrow aisles, then exploring a dark corner where a mysterious door lead to nowhere, and finally circling back to a creaky stairwell that swept upstairs to the forbidden balcony children so loved to explore when their parents weren't watching.

The sound of Cary's crutches thumping rhythmically against the long pine boards and creaky hollows was a welcome break after an hour of silence in this holy refuge, as well as a reminder to some that the path to truth could be both winding and simple, joyous yet difficult, innocent but also mysterious.

When Cary was three and one-half, Sue and Cathy decided to unlock his braces at the knees to increase his mobility. Suddenly he was able to climb small steps, hop over toys, and maneuver adroitly in tight spaces. Cary was fairly thrilled by his new freedom and quickly put it to use in his explorations of our backyard and the neighborhood.

Soon we were walking halfway down the block during our evening strolls. Then around the corner to check on Pirate, the funny black Labrador who galloped nervously from fence to fence. From there it was only a matter of time until we were hopping from stop sign to stop sign.

Some nights he circled the entire block on his own. Others he walked partway and I carried him the rest of the way on my back. Short or long, I could always count on Cary to point out some little bug or flower I overlooked, and then to ask me six questions about why it was there or whether it was dangerous. Later, I would hear him in his room quietly repeating what I said. It took awhile before I realized what he was up to. He was memorizing the information so the next time he could tell me instead of asking a question.

One night I heard Cary cooing in his darkened bedroom.

"Hey, what are you doing?" I said, peeking inside.

"Nothing."

"You're doing something."

"I'm just making a pretend dove sound," Cary said. "Coo de coo . . . coo de coo . . . coo de coo."

Earlier we had paused to listen to two doves hidden high in the trees fill the evening with their soft, murmuring exchange. "Coo de coo yourself," I said, chuckling. "Now go to sleep."

Months later, after we had moved to a new house, Cary gained still more freedom when one of the small stainless-steel bars locking his hips cracked, allowing him to bend and crouch at the waist instead of remaining rigid.

Ordinarily, we would have rushed to the brace shop for repairs. But Cary was due for a new set of braces in a few weeks. By the time the repairs were finished we would be ready to go back. We decided to let it go.

Cary was thrilled. Instead of walking in a stiff four-point gait, he could thrust himself up on his crutches and then swing his trunk and legs ahead, mimicking the motion of a pendulum. It didn't look pretty but it was a quicker and easier way of locomotion and helped him stick closer to the other children in the neighborhood and his classmates at school.

The new order of walking did not go by without prompting a small crisis in our household. We worried that we were risking long-term damage to Cary's knees and hips by not keeping him locked up. Rich Davidson was not encouraging. He thought Cary was slouching forward and that this was placing a major strain on his quadriceps. "While this crouching posture may be a quick way for him to get around, I think in the long run it is going to prove to be markedly energy-consuming," he observed in a report at the time.

A physical therapist at the new Pre-K program also was

critical of his new walking style. She insisted that it was important for children like Cary to stand as erectly as they could so they could greet their peers eye to eye and gain a sense of self-confidence.

Cathy and I went back and forth on the issue. One day we agreed with Davidson, only to find his approach narrow and one-sided the next. The problem was that the issue was not only medical. Our decision would also affect how Cary played and whether or not he could keep up with the other children. Many times doctors failed to take the social and psychological effects of their decisions into account. Trained in a clinical vacuum, they understood nerves or the brain or the heart, but not necessarily the patient.

In the end, we decided to leave Cary's hips and knees unlocked. No one could say with any degree of certainty that he would still be walking at fifteen, let alone thirty, if we held him to a rigid four-point gait. On the other hand, leaving his braces unlocked allowed Cary to move more freely and independently in a world that was already severely constrained.

As with most decisions, this one was neither clear nor faultless. We respected the others' opinions. But as parents we had to take the whole child into account and balance what we knew today against what we couldn't see in the future. Our reasoning evolved slowly and fitfully, fashioned more on intuition than intellect. Like any compromise, it was not made without fear.

ELEVEN

Growing Pains

Cary grew like a magic stalk during these early years, bending time and steel. One day he was a fuzzy infant encased in chalky ankle casts, the next a fearless little boy who had to be warned repeatedly to slow down. Although a picky eater who dined on pizza and chocolate milk, he ranked in the fiftieth percentile for height and the seventy-fifth percentile for weight for all children his age. Compared with children with spina bifida, who are shorter on average, Cary ranked even higher.

But this growth spurt had at least one unforeseen consequence. We had been told that a set of braces would last approximately two years. Cary outgrew his first pair in less than a year and has required a new set every year since then. Occasionally, Cathy managed to jury-rig a set with tape and wire so they lasted a few weeks longer. But even these economizing steps eventually foundered and we had to order a new pair.

In theory, this should have been a relatively painless process. Rich Davidson would give us a prescription. The orthotists would measure Cary and make a mold. And a few weeks later we would pick up the new pair—at a cost of $2,100 to our medical plan.

But with tensions increasing between insurers and providers, and soaring health-care costs a front-page story, even the simplest medical routines had a way of turning into bureaucratic passion plays and gut-wrenching negotiations.

The brace shop we used did not have a contract with our insurer, and management told us repeatedly that it had no intention of signing one. "Even if we had a contract, you would still have to pay cash for Cary's braces and submit the invoice to your insurer," a billing clerk informed us—well, not with relish, but with a certain zest. The shop's policy, which was unbending, required parents to pay twenty percent up front and the remaining eighty percent upon delivery of the braces.

"We don't have that kind of money," I advised the clerk, a painfully thin apparatchik with wandering eyes and a three-story hairdo. I doubted many other people did either.

"If you want you can talk to the manager," she replied coolly.

Rob Morgan was sympathetic but unmoved. "If I had to wait for the insurance companies to pay," he explained, "I would have gone broke years ago."

"What about the parents?" I said. "Is the idea that it's easier for us to go broke?"

Morgan frowned. "Believe me, I know how hard it is on some of my parents," he said. "But I'm running a business. Maybe if insurers paid me on time we wouldn't have this problem."

Morgan reserved special antipathy for HMOs, which he said demanded steep discounts and only covered a single set of braces, leaving parents, charities, and government programs to pick up the expense. "If it's left to me, I'll never do business with an HMO," he said.

I explained that our HMO had agreed to provide more than one set of braces for Cary, in writing no less, but Morgan didn't seem to listen, intimating that we must have received special treatment because I was a reporter.

"Yeah, we refused to take no for an answer and made dozens of phone calls," I shot back angrily.

In the first year alone we had written more than three dozen letters and had made more than fifty phone calls to our insurer, correcting mistakes, asking for guidance, and demanding services. It wasn't because we enjoyed these encounters; Lord knows we had better things to do with our time. We did it because we had no other choice. If Cary was going to get the best possible care, we had to lobby for him. Most parents give up the first time their insurer tells them *no* because they don't want the hassle. We couldn't afford such a laissez-faire attitude. We had to get involved and fight. Now, with a handful of words, Morgan had managed to dismiss all of our efforts.

Like many medical providers, Morgan also was prone to exaggerate the supposed evils of HMOs, which didn't just pay bills but also demanded a say in where and how medical care was given. Physicians and other caregivers viewed these intrusions as a violation of their traditional autonomy. But they also were concerned about the impact of prepaid health plans on their pocketbooks. HMOs' fixed, all-inclusive fees carried a financial risk for inefficient providers as well as put an end to the decades-old gravy train known as fee-for-service medicine.

To be sure, we had our share of insurance problems. Our HMO managed to flub numerous medical claims, especially the first year or two, triggering dunning notices from doctors, hospitals, and collection agencies. The tone of these letters varied from threatening to arrogant and caused us more headaches and work. "Final notice," one began. "If payment is not received in fourteen days, your account will be forwarded to a collection agency." Another letter chastised, "Keep in mind that the doctor does not have a contract with the insurance company . . . you do. It is your responsibility to see that they pay on time." We did the only thing we could—writing letters and making phone calls to correct the mistakes and speed up payment. It was annoying but after a while it also became rote.

From what I could see, it didn't matter what kind of insurance you had. These kind of hassles were the by-product of an industry slowly drowning in its own paperwork. Our HMO eventually assigned a mid-level manager to help coordinate Cary's numerous claims and smooth our way through the byzantine medical bureaucracy. If a claim got bounced back, I picked up the phone and called Debbie Heim, and most of the time she straightened it out. I didn't have to channel-surf my way through wave after wave of claims clerks until I finally stumbled onto the right one. This small step made all the difference.

More important, we had not been denied care, cast off to hacks and incompetents, or rigidly limited to a narrow band of medical providers, the way so many established physicians warned us we would be. In fact, we had been allowed to use doctors and hospitals that did not belong to our plan without any financial penalty. It had not been easy. We had to negotiate with our insurer each step of the way, but we usually found them willing to listen, if not always in agreement with us.

After several weeks of discussions, Morgan agreed to accept payment from our HMO. Why the change of heart? I could never figure that out. But it wasn't because he suddenly became a fan of HMOs. He continued to bad-mouth our plan every chance he had. Finally, we switched to another provider.

A physician friend who works as a public health officer once volunteered the following warning about HMOs. "You know, Gil, you and I both know HMOs don't do a good job with chronic illness. They're designed for taking care of Yuppies and healthy mothers, not children like your son."

"Tell me this," I replied, "what insurance plan is set up for chronically ill children?"

The telephone line suddenly grew quiet.

"Because if you know of one I wish you would let me in on the secret."

Steve dropped the subject and moved onto something a little more neutral, the plummeting fate of the Philadelphia Phillies.

In hindsight, I think we both know why.

The fact of the matter is that even in America, one of the wealthiest and best-insured nations in the world, there is no adequate health plan for the estimated 1.2 million children with severe illnesses and disabilities. Whether one belongs to an HMO, Blue Cross & Blue Shield, a commercial insurer, or one of dozens of other hybrid plans, the story is essentially the same. Important services and equipment aren't covered. Claims processing and paperwork are a nightmare. Communication between families and insurers is dodgy at best. Services are scattered. And families incur substantial out-of-pocket costs for deductibles, co-payments, and various ancillary services.

These days insurers talk a good game about managing the health of their subscribers. However, very few actually do this. What they really mean when they refer to managing care is negotiating prices and watching over doctors' shoulders to make certain they don't do too many tests or keep Grandma in the hospital an extra day. These steps save money. But they do little to help families put together a good, affordable network of caregivers.

How many insurers can honestly say that they have sat down with the family of a chronically ill child and their physicians to plot out an appropriate course of treatment?

Hold on there, I suspect some readers might say. What role does an insurer have in making medical decisions? What's to stop that insurer from choosing the least expensive doctors and hospitals? And who's to say I want to be locked into those decisions?

The fact is that insurers make these decisions all the time. You just don't see them. That's because they are made behind closed doors at the insurer's headquarters. They occur when a claim is reviewed for payment or a "prior approval" form is submitted for surgery. They take place in your doctor's office when the insurer visits to go over his practice patterns. They even occur in your workplace when your rates are raised by multiples of the consumer price index because somebody is using too many services.

Which would you prefer: that the insurer make these decisions for you, or that you have a say in the decisions affecting where and how your child will be cared for?

Another serious problem with health insurance is that it isn't portable. In plain English what this means is: you can't take it with you. Say I got a better offer from another newspaper. I would have to drop my present policy and accept whatever medical plan my new employer offered. If it happens to be a better policy—great, I luck out. But suppose it's not as good. Or suppose the new plan has a waiting period or preexisting condition clause, as commonly occurs, and Cary was excluded. Experience shows that I wouldn't be able to go out on my own and buy insurance for Cary because no company would accept him. In insurance terms, he's already a defined risk. I would be stuck between a rock and a hard place, in effect, a hostage to my current employer. As such, I would join the estimated one million other American families who currently face such a dilemma.

If money weren't involved, none of this would be a problem. However, big dollars are at stake. In April 1989, CDC researchers estimated that "annual medical and surgical care costs in the United States for all persons with spina bifida probably exceed $200 million." More recently, Duke University investigators reported that average medical costs for the first twenty years of life for a person with spina bifida were $240,000—or $12,000 a year. A significant portion of these expenses are front-loaded, that is, they are incurred shortly after birth. Afterward, they usually go down, then rise again whenever the child is hospitalized.

Our own experience mirrors these findings. I once estimated that the first year of Cary's life cost $50,000, with the vast bulk of that incurred during the first thirteen days of his life. Later on, there were the bills for straightening his clubfeet ($1,500 per foot for the surgeon), casting charges ($85 per foot), anesthesia ($450 for the doctor), spina bifida clinic ($300 per visit), follow-up office visits ($35 a visit), and various and sundry charges for X-rays, CT and MRI scans (ranging from $150 to $1,000). Our out-of-pocket costs have averaged between $1,500 to $3,500 annually, none of which is recoverable at tax time because our adjusted gross income is a little too high.

The best estimate of what it costs to care for all disabled and chronically ill children in America is twelve years old. A national survey in 1980 put the figure at about $1.5 billion dollars. The number has risen, but how much is anyone's guess. Paul Newacheck, a respected health economist who specializes in the area, told me it could be as high as $5 billion today.

That's a big number. However, its impact shrinks when placed in proper context. In 1990, Americans spent $650 billion on medical care. More than $100 billion alone was spent on the elderly by Medicare, the taxpayer-financed health plan for those over sixty-five. One-third of that $100 billion was spent during the last six months of life of Medicare beneficiaries, often when they were hooked up to an insulting array of breathing and feeding devices in the ICU.

Relative to the elderly then, who have already had an opportunity to savor many of life's important experiences—school, work, marriage, family, travel—we spend a fraction on our frailest and most vulnerable population. Not only does this seem unfair, it smacks of stinginess and distorted social policy.

It may be that nothing short of a full-blown national health insurance program will be able to redress such an imbalance in our medical spending. However, even though there is increased interest, such a radical departure from our existing public-private insurance system seems unlikely any time soon.

In the interim, insurers could move a long way toward easing the burden of families with severely ill children, improve the care of these kids, and possibly save themselves a few dollars if only they would view themselves as partners rather than as payers. Case management and coordination of benefits and services are not too much to ask for in 1991. Nor is it an especially radical notion to require insurers to pay for braces and crutches or a physical therapy session once a week. In the long run, everyone will benefit.

TWELVE

Under the Microscope

Cary was scrubbed clean and ready an hour before his bus arrived. His snack was packed (Yoo-Hoo and pretzel sticks) along with an extra diaper and spare set of clothes, per school instructions, in his sky blue backpack. For once, he had eaten without protest, his hair was neatly combed, and his teeth were brushed and sparkling.

"Daddy, is the bus almost here?" he asked for what had to be the fiftieth time this early September morning.

"No, Cary, not yet. I told you it won't be here until eight-thirty. Maybe even a little later."

He fell quiet then, tapping his fingers on his knee, framing the morning's events. "At eight-thirty the bus is coming for Malberg School. I think it's going to be bus number four. That's what I hope." Four was Cary Gaul's favorite number in the whole wide universe.

"Okay, picture time," I said, positioning Cary in front of our new house. I had chosen white knee-length shorts and a spiffy red Izod shirt, with the requisite alligator, for his first day of school. Cathy, who couldn't be here because she was teaching art at a local Friends school, had decorated Cary's crutches with different-colored tape. "Cary, you look like a million bucks," I said.

"Cheese," he said, sliding easily into a big smile.

The bus arrived closer to nine than eight-thirty, delayed by unusually heavy traffic. It was a stumpy version of the standard yellow school bus of childhood memory, with a special lift in the rear. As Cary quickly noted, it wasn't number four. But number eight was nearly as good and he didn't skip a beat, stepping on the lift and disappearing inside.

"At least someone is ready for school," Mrs. Nelson, the driver, said.

"You couldn't get here soon enough," I said.

My heart ached and soared at the same time. Cary had attended school in one form or another since he was seven months old. He had spent nearly three years at Kingsway, where he learned to walk, and another year in a three-year-old pre-K program in Haddon Township, where we lived until Cary was four. But this was different. During the summer, we had moved to Cherry Hill, and now Cary was starting a four-year-old Pre-K in the district where he would spend his school years and was just a year removed from kindergarten. This little boy who had given us such a fright was already slipping away from us. How much longer would it be before he had spun completely out of our protective grasp and was open to the world?

I followed Mrs. Nelson's bus to the Malberg School this first morning and secretly watched Cary from across the parking lot. I saw a happy child bounce off of the lift and quickly blend in with the other kids and teachers. Once one of the teachers reached down and gave Cary a friendly pat on the head and I imagined him chattering away about this and that, like he did in the friendly confines of his home. Just before he disappeared inside the school, I saw him add a little twist to his hop-step, his signature when he was excited, and my heart roared with pride. "You can do it," I whispered. "You can do it."

Driving home through the well-manicured neighborhoods of Cherry Hill, I couldn't help worrying about Cary. Would he like his teachers and classmates? Would they like him? Would they understand him when he bollixed his sentences and chattered on like a cocktail party patron or grow exasperated and walk away? Would they see the promise in him that we did or focus on his shortcomings? Most important, would he be happy and safe?

The answers would come later, of course. For now, Cary was still catching up to other children intellectually and socially, a leader in some skills, but clearly lagging in others.

This was perhaps the most frustrating aspect of spina bifida. Even though most of the children have normal intelligence, the vast majority suffer from learning problems that plague them academically and further stigmatize them socially.

The numbers are overwhelming. A 1980 study found

that between seventy and eighty percent of children with spina bifida exhibited "marked educational handicaps," requiring them to attend special education programs. Two subsequent reports estimated that between fifty to seventy-five percent of these children have learning disabilities that impeded their academic progress.

They have trouble learning to print and write because their fingers are floppy and weak. Their eyes don't track normally, skipping over columns of numbers, missing some rows entirely, reversing others. Although strong readers, they often have trouble remembering key points of stories and books. It isn't a question of vocabulary. They often have strong, rich, and expressive language. Yet they frequently have trouble retrieving the right word to express an idea. Frustrated, they resort to using the same words and phrases over and over, even though they are inappropriate. Organization, mathematical concepts, and problem solving pose intellectual mine fields for children with spina bifida because their brains don't "see" abstract problems the way a normal brain does. Alternatively, they may understand an idea but be unable to decode it and write it down on paper. Something gets lost in the translation, leaving their ideas scattered like marbles following a break.

Cary displayed symptoms of many of these problems. He could recall the smallest details about places we had visited months or even years before. Yet when asked to describe a movie he had just seen, he would have to stop and think hard about it. Even then his answers were usually sketchy.

Cary loved to read and learned this discipline on his own before he was five. However, he had trouble recalling even the most basic facts of stories unless he had memorized them.

"Where did Alice follow the White Rabbit?" I asked him one night while we were reading *Alice in Wonderland*.

"I don't know," Cary said.

"Think hard."

He did. Some nights I could practically hear the cells and neurons crackling inside of his head. Yet without prodding, Cary frequently had difficulty retrieving the information. That was fine now, when we had time, but what would happen in school when time was at a premium?

Cary's way of compensating was to talk about everything and anything except the question at hand. Instead of discussing the Rabbit's whereabouts, he would introduce a character from a television show or start talking about another book or a trip he had taken. If that didn't work, he would make up silly answers or bury his head in the pillow. When he was older and got a little more sophisticated about these things, he'd simply say, "I don't know" or "I'm not going to tell you."

But deep inside that beautiful brain of his, Cary must have understood. I say this because Cathy and I would frequently find him studying his books and practicing his answers.

"What are you doing, Cary?" we would gently ask.

"Oh, nothing," he would answer, embarrassed at being discovered.

If he liked a book or a tape, he would pour over it obsessively until he had committed every last detail to memory. In part, he was just doing something he enjoyed. However, it was also a way of compensating for his inability to express himself quickly. The drawback was that his language seemed stilted and even bizarre at times.

Instead of engaging someone normally in conversation, he would drag out the words and phrases he had memorized. It was so much simpler to live in this rigid but artificial world than face the real world, where spontaneity and verbal mobility were prerequisites to successful relationships.

Cary's obsessions also extended to real people. One year, he talked endlessly about a boy named Richie in his three-year-old pre-K class. Who is this Richie? we wondered. As it turned out, he was the biggest boy in the class, a boy who made funny faces and had a special laugh.

Then there was Chloe, a classmate of Greg and the daughter of a friend of ours. Cary absolutely idolized Chloe. If he knew he was going to see her on a particular day, he would talk about it constantly. But when the time actually arrived, Cary wouldn't know what to do with himself. "It's Chloe," he would sputter, prancing about excitedly on his toes but refusing to look. Why Chloe? And why this weird approach-avoidance behavior? We could never figure it out. Something about Chloe just tickled Cary's imagination, filling him with expectation, but also intimidating him a little.

Many of these marginal behaviors were like that—made of gauze and cotton and feather. Try as we might, we couldn't grasp them. Couldn't ascribe a rationale to them. They were neither here nor there. Neither so debilitating that Cary couldn't cope, nor so inconsequential that we didn't need to worry.

So much of his behavior was compensatory and masking. Verbally, Cary was a star, light years ahead of his peers. For this reason, he got along better with adults than with most children. They seemed to appreciate and delight in his verbal acuity. And yet his verbal skill was all window dressing, camouflage, and stealth. His words were like beautifully designed airplanes that plummeted to the ground soon after they were launched. They lacked controlling and steering mechanisms, and the wiring seemed wrong, spurting signals one moment, going blank the next.

Some researchers attribute the high incidence of learning problems among children with spina bifida to the fact that they are immobile during the critical first year or two of life, when perception, motor skills, and sensory integration are established in the brain's pathways. Others speculate it is because these children learn dependency from day one and live within an ever-tightening circle of family and friends. Some note that the brains of children with spina bifida are different anatomically from those of normal children and theorize that these malformations must interfere with the learning process. But how? Once more, I went looking for explanations that didn't seem to exist.

In spite of tremendous advances in recent years, scientists still do not know how the brain learns—at least not in any comprehensive sense. "We are just starting to look at some of these things," says neurosurgeon David G. McLone. "It is amazing how little we know.

"The important thing," McLone quickly adds, "isn't whether we know the cause. It's that we recognize the impact on the educational experiences of these children and take the necessary steps to help them. Keep in mind that twenty-five years ago virtually nothing was being done. Amazingly, we have come to a point where we are now worrying about schooling, independence, employment, and other long-term issues. Progress has been gradual but it has been significant."

McLone's comments bring to mind a number of

important points. One is the value of focusing on the strengths of disabled children, not on their weaknesses. Another is the evolving nature of the disease itself. Children born with spina bifida today are not the same as those born twenty, ten, or even five years ago. Advances in medicine and the gradual opening of society to the disabled have changed the profile of each successive generation, and will continue to do so. Lastly, it is all too easy to lump children with spina bifida or any other disabling condition into one big, monolithic pot. The truth is that these children are no different from the rest of us. Each is an individual, uniquely varied in his or her talents and abilities, a case study of the unusual riches of human biology.

When Cary was seven months old, Cathy started to bring him to an early intervention program at the non-profit Kingsway Learning Center in Haddon Township. There, under the watchful eyes of a child study team, he played with toys and puzzles, strung half-inch beads on a string, learned songs, built block towers, and experimented with computer games with Madge Bradley, the center's gentle and positive early childhood specialist.

Cary seemed to enjoy going to Kingsway. Even though he really didn't play with the other children, he liked being around them. You could see it in his eyes when he entered the narrow brick building and right away began looking for the other kids. When he saw someone he especially liked, his face would light up and he would nudge Cathy over in that direction.

The sessions at Kingsway were divided into five half-hour blocks and moved along quickly. During a typical afternoon, Cary might start off with Sue Cheney, the physical therapist, and work on a medicine ball, parallel bars, or standing in his crutches. Then it was on to the occupational therapist to practice fine motor skills like cutting with scissors or copying shapes with a crayon. Afterward, he moved on to Madge's room or down the hallway to the speech therapist. Each session ended with play time and a snack.

The atmosphere there was warm and supportive. Teachers were rarely patronizing and had lots of practical and useful information to share. Even so, the sessions were difficult at times. It was not pleasant having one's child under the microscope day in and day out. It wore us down, raising as many questions as it seemed to answer. To us, Cary seemed to make huge strides forward after a few years at Kingsway. But the staff measured his progress differently. For every gain, there was another problem or hurdle to overcome. That was the nature of their work. As professional observers, they were expected to study his every move. In many ways, it was an unreal atmosphere because Cary was an object as much as he was a person. All of the testing and measuring and judging, so temporal by nature, sometimes obscured how far our boy had come.

Following Kingsway, Cary moved on to a special Pre-K program for children with multiple handicaps run by our local school district in Haddon Township. Ordinarily, he would have been in a class with children his age. But the kids in the three-year-old class needed more help than Cary. So he was bumped up to a class with four-year-olds.

We worried that Cary would be in over his head with the older children. But as it turned out, our concerns were baseless. Cary kept up easily and blended in well with the other children. His teacher, Mary Ann Ogg, ran a structured program that managed to challenge the kids without overwhelming them. Each week, a child had a special job. One week it might be serving as the class weatherperson, the next turning out the lights at playtime. Cary took this latter task very seriously and actually taught himself how to balance on one crutch while using the other to reach up and snap off the light switch. "Watch this, Daddy," he surprised me one evening, turning off the kitchen light. I was properly impressed.

Mary Ann communicated with us on a daily basis via a spiral notebook we passed back and forth in Cary's backpack. If Cary had a particularly rough day, bumped himself, or had trouble with a task, we knew minutes after he got off the bus. Conversely, if he had a spectacular day, we could add our congratulations. The notebook was a deceptively simple way of communicating. And yet its simplicity was also its beauty. It cut through the bureaucracy and red tape and allowed us to keep our finger on the pulse of the situation without burdening the teachers with phone calls and extra meetings.

Surprisingly, few of Cary's other teachers have used a notebook to keep in touch. Those who have tried haven't had the staying power of Mary Ann. In most cases, the notebook has disappeared by Thanksgiving, only to resurface at the end of the year when Cary lugged home all of his belongings.

It wasn't our intention to overwhelm teachers and therapists with questions and information. However, in the course of a school year, there were things we needed to know and, frankly, they needed to know. Just because they were certified in special education didn't mean they were experts on spina bifida or the multitude of learning disabilities associated with it. In fact, most of Cary's teachers knew little about his condition and had only taught a small number of children with it during their entire careers. When Cary transferred into the Cherry Hill school district in 1990, he was the only child with spina bifida in the Malberg School program and one of only two children with the condition in the entire district. For that reason alone, we thought it was important to share information with his teachers.

Most of them welcomed this input. Some, like Lenore Weiner and Susan Baskies, Cary's physical and speech therapists, sought out information and made us feel like partners. For that we were grateful. On the other hand, a small number of teachers and consultants seemed to be fixed on reducing Cary (and the other children) to a formula. One incident in particular sticks in our minds. It occurred after we had moved to Cherry Hill at the end of his first school year.

Under federal law, teachers and learning consultants must sit down with parents each year to draft an Individualized Education Program, or IEP, for children in special education programs. A contract, enforceable in court, the IEP serves as the game plan for the upcoming year and contains a mixture of specific information (for example, the number of physical therapy sessions a child will receive each week) and more general goals having to do with behavior and education.

During one such session, Cathy noticed that under Behavioral Goals, a consultant had checked: "To learn to identify, accept, and to function within the limits of one's own strengths and weaknesses."

A warning bell sounded in the back of her brain. What does that mean? she inquired.

Mrs. Sparks, tall and self-assured, started to explain

how important it was for children with physical disabilities like Cary's to come to terms with their limits.

"Excuse me," Cathy interrupted. "I thought the purpose of school was to help Cary achieve his potential, not to set limits on what he can and cannot do. Don't you think he'll face enough obstacles in his life without teachers telling him he can't do certain things?"

Mrs. Sparks held her ground. Nobody was talking about setting limits, she insisted. Cary could try anything or do anything. His teachers certainly weren't going to hold him back.

"Maybe not explicitly," Cathy responded without flinching, "but it sure sounds like you don't expect much for him. Isn't it a little early to be lowering expectations?"

"Mrs. Gaul, no one is talking about lowering their expectations for Cary."

"Well, then, I guess I'm confused," Cathy said, "because that's what it sounds like."

In the end, Mrs. Sparks brushed Cathy's concerns aside by agreeing to pencil in a more appropriate goal. However, before the session was finished, she managed to lob one more psychological bomb at her corner.

A school psychologist had recently spent twenty minutes with Cary as part of the IEP evaluation and prepared a brief report. Among his findings, Mrs. Sparks explained, was that Cary exhibited signs of anger and sadness, which he was repressing.

Cathy was speechless. "Are you sure he's talking about Cary?" she finally managed to ask.

Yes, Mrs. Sparks replied. She hastened to add that none of the members of the child study team had actually spoken with the psychologist about Cary.

Cathy looked around the table. Some of Cary's teachers

also appeared dumbstruck. And with good reason: their reports uniformly described him as a happy, energetic, friendly child. In dozens of reports compiled over five years, no one had so much as hinted that Cary might be anything but happy.

"I can't believe this," Cathy said.

Later that evening, when I learned about the report, I didn't know whether to laugh or to cry. How anyone could presume to label another human being angry or sad on the basis of a twenty-minute interview was beyond me. "Did you see a copy of the report?" I asked.

"No. They didn't have one there. They said it was still being typed. And when I pressed her, Sparks didn't want to go into it in any great detail. She seemed to be on a really tight schedule and was just giving me the highlights," Cathy said.

"You mean lowlights."

"Right."

It took us months to get a copy of the report, although I don't think because of any dishonest intentions. It just seemed to get lost in the bureaucracy of the school district. As it turned out, in her rush, Mrs. Sparks had mischaracterized its findings.

"Interview, observations, and projective testing indicate that there is no evidence of serious emotional disorder," the psychologist wrote. "Like many children with physical handicaps involving ambulation, etc., Cary tends to emphasize the intellectual and thinking aspects of himself. There are positive feelings about school and an apparent interest in many areas of activity. There is some understandable sadness and lowering of self-esteem when he is unable to do things that he wants to do. This is quite common among children with spina bifida or other physical difficulties. Cary certainly shows strength in his ability to compensate for his areas of weakness, and he seems to derive a good deal of self-esteem from his good verbal skills and his ability to relate to others in an outgoing way."

"That doesn't sound like an angry or depressed child to me," I said to Cathy.

"Something got lost in the translation," she said, being generous. "What I wonder is how many other times it happens."

Too many, I'm sure. Surprisingly, my response wasn't anger so much as regret. I thought about the special power and authority all of these consultants hold over the lives of children like Cary, and how sad and tragic it must be to dismiss a child with a cliché. The shame of our educational bureaucracy is not its stultifying adherence to crushing regulations. It is the inability of its masters and practitioners to trust their own instincts. Confronted with information that flies in the face of reality, they opt for safety over truth and experience. If children are lost in the process, so be it.

THIRTEEN
The Drill

The summer before Cary started kindergarten we decided to take one more stab at resolving the nagging question of his dislocated hips.

Thus far, we had visited three out of five pediatric specialty clinics in the area, where we had received three different opinions. A fourth clinic didn't have a contract with our insurer. That left the Shriners Hospital in Northeast Philadelphia, one of twenty-three orthopedic and burn centers for children operated nationally by the Tampa-based charity and social organization.

We had heard mixed opinions about the rambling stone hospital just off busy Roosevelt Boulevard. Some parents raved about the warm atmosphere there and the attentive staff. Others complained that the hospital was set up like a charity ward from the twenties. But by this point we were less concerned with ambiance than with finding someone who could help us sort through this perplexing medical question.

We ended up seeing three different surgeons at Shriners. Two recommended operating to stabilize the hips. The third said toss a coin. But in any event, he could not guarantee Cary would be better off if he had the surgery. Nor could he promise the hips would remain in their jury-rigged sockets.

"Which means another operation," I said.

"Unfortunately, that's right."

"Not to mention another eight weeks immobilized in a body cast," Cathy pointed out.

"Probably more like six weeks," Dr. Fisher corrected her. "I like to get the kids standing in their braces as soon as I can. But you're right, it's a significant chunk of time."

"Well, what do you think?" Cathy asked as soon as we had stepped outside again.

"You want the truth?"

"Yup."

"I don't think we're any farther along today than we were three years ago. None of these guys has said it's going to make a big difference in the way he walks or how long he walks. All they've told us is maybe it will help avoid arthritis twenty or thirty years from now."

"If someone could tell me Cary would still be walking then, I might do it. But they can't. They have no way of knowing," Cathy said. "I want someone to tell me it's going to make Cary a stronger walker *now*. And nobody's able to say that."

"Is it worth having Cary operated on and in a body cast for six or eight weeks?"

Cathy shook her head. "I don't think it's fair to him. If it was going to make a difference, I'd say, definitely, let's do it. But right now it doesn't seem worth it."

Oddly enough, even while we were being encircled by disappointment, a great burden lifted from our shoulders. Perhaps in a year or two we would feel differently, maybe even revisit the issue. But for now the sheer uncertainty had won out.

Truth be told, we had another motive for going to Shriners.

Several parents had told us about an extraordinary physical therapist who worked there. Bright, energetic, and innovative, Peg Kelly was willing to try new approaches and keep working at difficult problems long after most therapists had surrendered. One mother phoned Cathy regularly to report on her daughter's progress. Carolyn had been in a body cast for months following hip surgery and had been having an especially tough time of it. Step by step, Peg had brought her back, and now she was walking better than ever.

As parents, you never know whom to believe. One parent's idea of a saint often turns out to be another parent's Therapist-from-Hell. It all depends on your expectations. Then again parents have been known to exaggerate their children's progress. That doesn't change just because a child is disabled. In fact, the competition may be more intense because the stakes are higher. We weren't immune from these pressures. Like other parents, we were constantly searching for that one doctor, therapist, or teacher who would make a difference in our child's life.

And so, on a brutally hot July afternoon, Cathy and Cary drove out to Shriners to meet with Peg Kelly. Ostensibly, the purpose of the visit was to see if Cary could get by without the bulky pelvic band that connected the two legs of his braces. With his hips unlocked, it didn't seem as though the band served much purpose, and it was heavy and cumbersome, especially when changing pants or diapers. Psychologically, we reasoned, it would be a big boost if the band could be removed without hurting Cary's gait or posture.

Peg Kelly met Cathy and Cary outside of the physical therapy room on the hospital's second floor. "Just a second," she said. "I'm going to call Karl up from the brace shop. I want him to watch Cary walk, too."

Unlike most children's hospitals, Shriners has its own in-house brace shop, where modern-day craftsmen like Karl Reebuck take ragged plaster molds and create exquisitely designed braces made of leather, plastic, steel, and carbide. As with all of the care at Shriners, one of the last true charity hospitals in America, there is no charge.

Peg and Carl removed the pelvic band from Cary's braces and then put him on a set of parallel bars with his knees locked to see if he could walk in a four-point gait. After several trips up and back, with no apparent problems, Peg gave Cary his crutches back and asked him to walk around the room. This time she attached a long thin belt around his waist and stood behind him in case he stumbled.

"How much are you helping him with the belt?" Cathy asked after Cary had hiked back and forth several times.

"I'm not holding him at all," Peg replied.

"Really?"

"He's doing it all himself."

Cary, realizing he was being praised, did a little dance.

"He really is doing a nice job," Karl said. "His hips aren't rocking back and forth at all."

"I think he's doing great," Peg said, studying Cary now. "His feet are pointing out a little, but it's not a big problem."

"So you think he might be able to get by without the band?" Cathy cautiously inquired.

"I don't see why not. He's a little wobbly. But that's just because he isn't used to it. He's not unstable or anything," Peg said.

Cathy couldn't believe it. Cary needed less of something, not more! Instead of adding to his braces, they were actually going to cut them down. Ever since he had received his first set, four years earlier, she had hoped that one day this would be possible. Now she had to convince herself that it was real. "What about his hips? Won't it be dangerous if he hasn't had hip surgery?" she asked.

Peg thought the question over for a minute. "It shouldn't make a difference unless he's unstable," she said. "We can always put him back in higher bracing if we need to."

Peg removed Cary's braces and bent his legs up and down. "When I push against this leg, I want you to pull this other leg up as hard as you can, okay, Cary?" she said. This simple test would give Peg an idea of the strength of Cary's quadricep muscles, which are crucial for walking. As children in braces grow and put on weight, these large, bulky muscles in the front of the thigh bear the brunt of the increased workload. Without strong quads, most disabled children have trouble walking and switch over to wheelchairs.

"They're not the strongest," Peg said, finishing up her

tests. "But they're not weak. The left leg seems a little stronger than the right."

"It's been that way since he was a baby," Cathy said.

"It's not that unusual."

The rest of the session was spent taking measurements for a new set of braces. Unlike Cary's present pair, the legs would be separate, and there would be no connecting pelvic band.

That night Cathy and the boys descended on me before I was even through the door.

"Dad, Dad, Dad, guess what?" Greg called excitedly. "Cary got his braces lowered today."

I looked at Cathy, who was smiling, then at Cary, who was dancing happily on his tiptoes.

"You're kidding."

"Look, no pelvic band," Cathy said, snapping the waistband of Cary's powder blue shorts.

"I can't believe it," I said.

"Guess what else, Daddy? I'm going to have blue braces," Cary said.

"Blue braces?"

"They're making Cary a new set of braces and he gets to pick out the color. He wants sky blue," Cathy explained.

As Cathy debriefed me, it quickly became clear that the trip to Shriners had been an extraordinary couple of hours.

"Gil, I can't tell you how nice it was to watch Peg Kelly and Karl working together. You know, that was the first time in five years that members of two different specialties actually looked at Cary at the same time. I was so impressed."

Subsequent trips buttressed these impressions. Peg and Karl were those rare exceptions in a system that often baffles parents and leaves them dispirited. Quick-witted and innovative, they were committed to the children and their work, which after all was the heart of the matter. There wasn't a phony bone in either of them.

A week later, Cathy and Cary returned to the brace shop at Shriners for a fitting. An older boy, maybe seventeen, with hawklike eyes and a stubby crew cut was also there being fitted for a prosthesis. By the sour look on his face, he was not pleased with the tan, rubber sleeve he was being shown.

"You don't happen to have any of these things in different colors?" he shyly inquired.

"As a matter of fact we do," the tech who was helping him said. A minute or two later he reappeared dangling a neon yellow sleeve.

The boy's face lit up. "That's awesome," he exclaimed. "Can I keep it if it fits?"

"Absolutely," the tech replied. "Let's try her out."

The boy stiff-legged his way around the room, gradually easing into a near-normal gait. "It feels good," he said.

Randy, the orthotist, smiled at his mother, a short, painfully thin woman, who nodded approvingly.

"It's probably a pretty small thing to you or me," Karl observed, "but to these kids, it is so important to fit in. They're already different. The last thing they need is to look nerdy or uncool."

It made sense. And yet this was the first brace shop we had encountered that offered kids a choice of colors and actually encouraged them to shine. The others constructed perfectly good braces but overlooked that braces were more than medical equipment. They were also clothing for disabled children, especially during warmer months when the kids were in shorts.

When it came time, Cary chose light blue braces with hot blue velcro straps. Another little girl who was there selected pink braces with neon pink velcro straps. Pink was Cary's second favorite color.

"Hey, look, Mommy," he said as Cathy and he were leaving. "That little girl has pink braces. Those are cool."

Cathy smiled at the girl's mother. "Yes, they are," she said.

"I really like pink," Cary said admiringly. "But I love blue. Blue is my favorite color."

At the age of five, Cary was more agile than ever. In no time at all, he was climbing short flights of stairs, hopping on and off adult-sized chairs, and stepping up into his school bus without assistance.

His already-ample confidence swelled. Cary was convinced he could do anything and go anywhere without our help. And he seemed bound and determined to prove it at every turn. He shooed away our pesky attempts to open doors for him and scolded me like a blue jay if I tried to help him in or out of the car.

"No, Daddy, I want to do it myself."

"Okay, okay, I was just trying to help."

"I don't need any help."

"I'm sorry."

"Watch me do it."

Cary had figured out how to lift himself up onto the seat with his crutches, wedge himself into a comfortable position, and put his seatbelt on all by himself. "Ready," he said upon finishing, in a tone that suggested there was never any question.

Cathy and I marveled at our little boy's ferocious need to

be independent, while trying to make sure he didn't hurt himself or become too pushy.

It wasn't an easy balance to strike, in part, because we were reluctant to hold Cary back, but also because he was such a physical child, who loved to join in the other kids' games, and had a hard time understanding when he couldn't keep up.

No amount of reasoning helped. Once he got it in his head that he wanted to do something, there was no holding him back. Our only hope was to divert his attention to something else, or let him try, knowing full well that heartache and crocodile tears would follow.

A good example of this was a small tree in our neighbor's front yard, which some of the little boys liked to climb. One day, when he was four, Cary saw several of the boys sitting in the lower branches and insisted on joining them. Nothing would placate him. He just had to climb that tree and be with the guys.

I finally gave in and escorted him over. "Hmmm," he said, eyeing the slick trunk. "How am I going to do this?" He wrapped his little arms around the trunk and tried to pull himself up. He tried to jump up and grab one of the low-lying branches. He even kicked the tree, hoping, I suppose, that it would magically transport him up there. When he realized nothing would work, he started to sob.

I lifted Cary up and sat him on one of the lower branches, and that stopped the tears. Even then I had to stand behind him with my hand on his back because his balance was so precarious. When he got down a few minutes later, he smiled at me and said, "That was fun." But I couldn't help noting that he never asked me to haul him back up in the tree. These days, when the neighborhood kids are sitting up there, he is content to dance around the trunk or poke one of his crutches up into the lower branches, as though that somehow connects him to the fun. I view this as a positive way of coming to terms with his handicap, and yet find myself quietly mourning for Cary, and what he has lost.

In the last year, some of the other neighborhood children have started to pay more attention to Cary's physical shortcomings. A few have even stopped playing with him because of them. They haven't said anything, at least not while we were within earshot, but they ran away or hid whenever Cary approached. At first, Cary's feelings were hurt. He wandered home sobbing that the kids were being mean to him. But after a while, the tears stopped. He spent more time by himself or asked Cathy to invite one of his other friends over to our house. One on one, Cary did just fine, even with the children who were mean to him as part of a group, which leads me to believe there was something else going on, some group dynamic that we weren't privy to. It may be as simple as Cary can't keep up when they play ball or sprint from house to house. They don't like waiting for him or the way it slows down their games. I don't blame them. But the fact that they have reasons doesn't make it any easier. There is nothing quite as lonely or painful as watching your child rejected. It is a terrifying feeling that rips apart all pretenses of order and well-being, rendering one brittle and afraid.

Fortunately, Cary is such an active, athletic little boy, that a setback here and there isn't going to leave his spirit permanently bruised. Athletic? Absolutely. I do not hesitate to use that word when describing my son. Cary loves to mix it up with his dad and brother, is surprisingly quick and agile, and possesses astounding stamina.

Anyone who spends a day with Cary discovers this

quickly enough. From the moment he bounces out of bed and crawls downstairs until he is finally asleep, he rarely stops. "I don't know how he does it," says his grandmother, Jane Candy, after a day together. "He's like that commercial on TV for the battery; he keeps going and going and going."

In the pool, where he is more or less on equal footing with other children, Cary shines. While many little boys his age still cling tightly to their mothers and fathers, Cary paddles happily from wall to wall, dives to the bottom to check for crocodiles, and loves to roughhouse with Gregory and me.

"Throw me over your shoulder like you do Gregory," he begs in the middle of these battles. Then, surfacing after a good dunking, he will cry: "Do it again, Daddy. Only this time turn me upside down so I make a bigger splash."

If possible, Cary is probably a little too brave and a little too innocent. He will ask for help, but only if he can't do something for himself. He is aware of his physical shortcomings but does not let them get in his way. All of which is admirable, and an attitude we hope he maintains throughout life, yet this leaves him vulnerable to questions and comments from other children.

In the fall of 1991, Cathy developed a little routine she refers to as "the spina bifida drill" just so Cary wouldn't be tongue-tied when other kids asked him about his braces and crutches. It goes something like this:

Cathy: "Hey, little boy, what's wrong with your legs?"
Cary: "I have spina bifida."
Cathy: "What's that?"
Cary: "It makes my muscles weak."
Cathy: "Why do you have those braces?"
Cary: "So I can walk."

Cathy: "Well, why do you have those crutches?"

Cary: "So I don't fall down."

The two of them practice the drill at odd moments—in the car, walking outside, at the store. Although Cary considers it a nuisance, he has committed the answers to memory. I know because I have overheard him confidently using them with strange children.

Would we be better off leaving Cary to fend for himself? The way we figure it, he's already doing that in spades, and will be doing it for the rest of his life. Cathy's clever routine is a small way of making Cary's journey a little bit easier. It is practical, direct, and effective. The handiwork of a skillful teacher.

FOURTEEN

Light One Candle

*Better to light one candle than curse
the darkness.*
—AN OLD QUAKER SAYING

Little by little, we watched
Cary reach out to other children. His need to be in control
was slowly subsumed by his desire to be included in the
neighborhood games, and his quirky obsessions gave way
to more creative and social play. Although still lagging
behind other children his age, he had clearly hurdled some
invisible block and was moving ahead.

This was especially evident when Cary was plopped into

unfamilar settings with children he didn't know. Before, he would have fussed and insisted that the other kids play one of his games, or else have wandered off by himself. Now he was much more flexible and willing to compromise.

One occasion in particular comes to mind. Cathy and Cary were visiting a local farmstead in search of interesting crafts. There, Cary encountered two other little boys who were playing pirates. Having already memorized the story of *Peter Pan*, he asked if he could join their game, only to be brushed off by one of the boys. "We're the captains and there can be only two captains," he exclaimed.

Instead of stalking off, crying, or insisting on being the only captain, Cary thoughtfully replied, "That's okay, there can be three captains. Then we can all play together and be friends."

The other little boy was so taken aback by his response, that he quickly invited Cary into their game. The newly formed trio played happily until it was time to go.

In the structured environment of school, where Cary was expected to do certain things and didn't have his parents to rescue him, he did just fine. The reports from his teachers and consultants emphasized how much he had matured socially in a short time.

"He really seems to have grown up a lot over the summer," Susan Baskies, Cary's speech teacher, told us during Back to School Night in the fall of 1991. "He's doing so well academically, and he really seems to fit in with the other children in his class."

"He's just much more focused this year," added Lenore Weiner, his physical therapist at Malberg School. "The only time I have a bit of difficulty is when he has to leave class. He doesn't like to miss out on anything, which is good, of course, because it shows how much he enjoys school."

Cary's growing attachment to his classmates and teachers also appeared in a learning consultant's report prepared about this time. Apparently Cary had put up a fuss when the woman came to get him for some testing, refusing to answer her questions until she promised to take him back.

"The fact that he was concerned about having sufficient play time with classmates was a truly positive indication that he has developed strong relationships with them," she later wrote.

"He is less egocentric and less inclined to relate solely to adults. He wants to be part of the group," another consultant noted in a report.

Cary seemed to have no trouble making friends at school and brought home an ever-expanding list of buddies. We took advantage of these friendships to invite classmates over on weekends and after school. Cary and his buddies dug in our sandbox, played with cars, roamed the backyard in search of tigers and bears, and moved easily between our garage, which was crowded with boxes of toys, and our family room, where there was a VCR and Disney tapes.

"I can't tell you how nice it is to see Cary playing normally with another child," Cathy called to report during one of these initial visits. "There's been no fighting or fussing or tears. Nobody's run away. The boys have played together happily for two entire hours. In fact, they've been so quiet, I've hardly known they were here."

As the months slipped by and another school year started up, a few of the neighborhood boys also began to drop by after school to play with Cary. We were delighted. Safely settled in our house, they seemed to do just fine together. It wasn't until the games moved outside, and the kids started to run from house to house, that Cary was left behind—literally and figuratively.

No one had a better view of Cary's progress than Cathy. She spent the most time with him and understood the dynamics of neighborhood play far better than I. Thus, after months and months of worrying, I was encouraged to hear her say one fall afternoon that Cary was doing better.

"He's getting there. I can really see him trying. He's playing with the other kids better and there's a whole lot less of those bizarre little behaviors. He's still not where he should be for his age, but he's not nearly as far behind as he was. I think he just needs a little more time."

It is our hope that after the other children have slowed down a little, they will see in Cary the same positive traits we admire and enjoy. His warm, outgoing personality. His curiosity and enthusiasm for things small and large. His terrific sense of humor and love of play. His big, tender heart and loyal instincts. And his tremendous inner strength and courage.

Cary was also beginning to bloom intellectually.

Each day, he seemed a little more aware of the world around him and how it worked. His grasp of complex ideas and relationships, while still lagging, was also growing. This was reflected in the questions he asked us, which were sharper and increasingly complicated. No longer content with the who, what, and where of things, Cary now wanted to know *why*.

Why couldn't he go out after dark in the backyard? Why did the recycling truck come on Thursdays but not on Mondays? Why didn't he go to school on weekends? Why did Gregory play soccer and he didn't? And why couldn't he eat pizza every night for supper if that was what he liked?

Years before, when Gregory was three, we had dubbed him the "Why Monster" because his response to everything was "Why?" It had taken him a little longer, but now Cary had taken over the title. Instead of being exasperated, we were tickled. Cary was growing before our eyes.

One morning, Cary announced at breakfast that he didn't want to die.

"You're not going to die," we reassured him, "you've got your whole life to live."

"Well, why do people die?"

"Usually they get old and their bodies get tired," Cathy said.

"But why do they die?" Cary persisted. "Why do their bodies get tired?"

"Their bodies just stop going forward and start going backward."

"I don't want to go backward. I want to go forward."

"You are, for a very long time," I said.

Cary thought about that while he gulped down a spoonful of cereal. "When I die," he continued, "will I come back as a baby, like Jana?" Jana was his one-year-old cousin from Florida, whom both of the boys loved dearly.

"No, you won't come back as a baby," Cathy said matter-of-factly.

"Well, when I come back," Cary said, "I'm going to be a boy. A boy named Cary."

Another night, Cary and I were lying in his bed when he said he planned to get up at seven A.M.

"Why so early?" I asked.

"Because that's when 'Mr. Wizard' is on."

"You watch 'Mr. Wizard'?" I asked dubiously.

"Um-hmmm."

"Do you understand it?"

"Yes," Cary replied in a tone that suggested, "Doesn't everybody?"

Still doubtful, I asked, "What is 'Mr. Wizard' about?"

Cary shuffled his blankets. "It's about doing stuff," he said.

Which was exactly right. Mr. Wizard, the popular TV tinkerer, used everyday objects as his props to poke around the edges of science. "Okay," I said, "I'll see you and Mr. Wizard tomorrow morning."

Cary was beginning to *get* things. And not just facts or words that he could commit to memory. A sense of awareness and consciousness was exploding deep inside his brain, giving rise to a more creative and critical thinker.

In attempting to explain this phenomenon to others, I have taken to using an admittedly imprecise analogy. The way most kids learn things, I said, is like flicking on a light switch. You hit the button and the light comes on. With Cary, it's more like using a dimmer switch. The light increases gradually, starting from a small pale circle and slowly rising to a bright pool of light. The end result is the same. It just takes longer.

Similarly, there was no one day or week or month, or even year, for that matter, that we could point to and say, this is when Cary started to change, this is when he went from being a bright but self-absorbed child to a responsive, engaging little boy of promise.

The process was much less certain that than, much more subtle and amorphous, occurring over hundreds of days, during thousands of small and large moments that often were invisible to the human eye, and continues even as I write.

By the age of five and a half, Cary picked up most factual subject matter quickly and easily. He read books like *The Ox Cart Man* and *Peter Pan* without prompting, taught himself many of the state capitals by playing with a magnetic map, and possessed an ever-expanding vocabulary.

His fine motor skills were also coming along, although more slowly. He still had trouble making a pencil and crayon do what he wanted. His floppy fingers tended to fly away from rulered lines without warning, giving rise to a mishmash of mischievous squiggles. And he continued to have a difficult time transferring some things he clearly understood onto paper—numbers being a perfect example.

"Practice at home," Cary's kindergarten teacher, Mrs. DeLuca, wrote on the top of the mimeographs he brought home. And practice he did. Ensconced at the kitchen table after supper, Cary crafted row after row of looping S's and curling 3's, without so much as a whimper, until he got them just right.

Before he entered kindergarten in the fall of 1991, Cary was given the Kaufman Assessment Battery for Children, a test for factual knowledge and skills in the areas of reading, arithmetic, language, and riddles. His mean score of 118 ranked in the above-average category. Not surprisingly, he tested strongest in reading skills and weakest in riddles, which required him to infer abstract verbal concepts from a series of clues.

Cary answered nine riddles correctly, scoring in the fifty-third percentile of all children, or roughly equivalent to what might be expected for his age at the time—five years and three months. But I was encouraged that even his mistakes hinted at a growing sense of awareness.

For instance, when the person administering the test asked Cary, "What is made of rubber, pops, and floats in the air?" he responded airplane instead of balloon. Not a completely inappropriate guess.

When asked the profession of former heavyweight champ, Mohammed Ali, Cary answered, "Wrestlemania." Again, he wasn't that far off the mark, especially when you consider that Cary had never seen the popular boxer before, but did watch wrestling on television from time to time with his brother.

During still another test, Cary was asked to draw a picture of a man. He proceeded to sketch your classic stick figure with an oval head, narrow trunk, and long A-frame legs. "Interestingly," the consultant wrote, "Cary drew a brace on his picture of a man."

Unfortunately, she stopped without explaining why this was interesting. That was left to us to interpret. Did Cary think everyone wore braces? Or was he drawing a picture of himself, in which case this might be seen as a positive, even healthy sign, the stirrings of self-awareness?

I opted for the latter. It just made more sense. Even as Cary was reaching out to the world, trying so hard to fit in, he also was discovering himself. These two events were mirror images of the same process of self-discovery. Here, in a simple drawing of a stick figure, was the first outward expression of how Cary saw himself. As such, it was a remarkable and terrifying moment.

Years from now, the issues will be far more complicated and potentially devastating than those we face today. What then? Will the image Cary sketches for himself be bold and strong, a survivor, in the best sense of the word, able to rise above trauma and uncertainty to embrace life? Or will he draw himself as a cripple, hobbled by braces, unable to keep up, as someone who knows only life's bruises and cruel twists?

Part of me wishes I could see ahead so I would know what to look out for, which steps to take now to prepare and protect our son, what obstacles to avoid. But I know this is impossible. And just as assuredly as we are starting to let go of Gregory, we will one day let go of Cary. He will stand or fall on his own, enticed and challenged by the rituals most of us take for granted, dating, sports, college, work, marriage, sex, independence, family. None of these issues will ever be as simple. But perhaps they will be simpler than I now imagine.

Searching the past for clues is of little help. Most medical literature is hopelessly outdated or simply nonexistent. Considering that virtually everything important known about spina bifida has been learned in the last three decades, this is hardly surprising, although of little comfort. The therapeutic nihilism of the fifties and sixties has given rise to a condition that lacks history or context in the nineties. Medicine alone must bear that shameful mark.

The good news is that a small but hardy band of researchers is working diligently today to unravel some of the long-ignored mysteries of this baffling and horrific condition. It is entirely possible that the next thirty years will see the genetic underpinnings and environmental triggers of spina bifida uncovered, as well as significant advances in its treatment. We are grateful for these efforts.

Their corollary, however, is that the future of spina bifida is being rewritten yearly, if not monthly. More is known today about Chiari II malformations, tethered cord syndrome, and renal failure due to reflux than ever before. The work of Donald Lollar in Atlanta, and other researchers, is also beginning to provide valuable insights into the causes and treatment of learning disabilities associated with spina bifida. As a result, each new generation of children stands to fare a little better than the one before it. So, too, will the issues they confront be different.

I had to remind myself of this frequently while working on this book. Time and time again, I encountered researchers and doctors depressed by the failure of this generation of young adults with spina bifida to achieve independence. This perspective was best expressed by Donald Riegel, the dedicated Pittsburgh neurosurgeon.

"What we're seeing," Riegel told me during a visit, "is that at the point these young adults should be separating and moving into society, many of them are coming back home. They aren't achieving independence or thriving the way we hoped they would."

There are any number of explanations for this. While the development of shunts and surgical techniques to close the lesions of newborns dramatically increased survival rates, they did not magically wipe the slate clean. Shunt revisions and other complications were legion in these earlier populations. In addition, as we noted earlier, advances in chronic care have lagged, giving rise to a host of secondary medical problems that greatly interfere with daily activities of living.

Thirty years ago, there were no early-intervention programs to provide infants and parents with critical services like physical and occupational therapy. Twenty years ago, there were no federal laws ensuring disabled children a meaningful education. And as recently as five years ago, there was no American Disabilities Act to protect the civil rights of the disabled in the workplace and public settings.

All of which begs the question of how meaningful it is to draw hard and fast conclusions from this first group of survivors. The lessons of the past have to do with indifference and neglect and are cautionary rather than descriptive or revealing. The battles of the disabled generally, and families visited by spina bifida specifically, are still being fought today on numerous fronts and will continue to be waged for many years to come.

"I am embarrassed to say that we are only getting started," says one prominent physician-researcher who requested anonymity because of his ties to a large university-based program. "As long as this condition has been around, we have barely scratched the surface. I am not proud of that. I understand how it came to pass. But I do not feel especially good about it. And if I were a parent, I think I might be more than a little embittered."

But what good will bitterness do? It won't help fix Cary's hips or make him continent. It can't solve the learning disabilities he suffers from or ease his path socially through the neighborhood or at school. Only progress and caring can do that. And bitterness just gets in the way of those.

Whether he is comfortable in the role or not, Cary will be a trailblazer, no less daring or courageous than any other explorer, pushing against boundaries and expanding horizons as he searches for his place in life. And we will be his advocates, pressuring his doctors and teachers and insurers when they need to be pressured, and stepping aside when they don't.

We know it will never be easy. But then how could it

be? Chronic disease is a formidable opponent, malevolent, ruthless, and tyrannical in its pursuit of victims. Its path is rarely straight, and there are few ablutions and epiphanies along the way. Irony and false starts mark its long march. So, too, pain and frustration and suffering.

All we can ask is that our son gets a fair chance. That in a society that measures its margin of compassion in tax-exempt vouchers and Labor Day telethons, there is a room, a corner, a pew, or a heart for Cary, where he might be comfortable and welcome.

Every so often, when we are full of worry about the future, Cary will remind us with a look or a word that he is more than a complicated medical history or perplexing educational report. He is a child, a person, foremost, full of mischief and wonder and fun, one who is gifted with the rare ability to make others laugh; a boy blessed with a good and trusting heart. Cary's life cannot be separated from illness. But his life is not about illness. It is about courage and promise, and most of all, it is about love. For above all, Cary possesses the gift of loving, and that is more rewarding and magical and reaching than all of the other gifts combined.

EPILOGUE

Ghosts in the Graveyard

I was thinking of you today while on the train to Philadelphia, wondering what it would be like a few years from now when you realize what it means to have spina bifida, and whether that knowledge would come to you all at once or build slowly over time, like a rain-swollen river finally taking its banks.

I closed my eyes and a powerful image rose up in front of me.

In it, I was arguing with God, scolding Him for being cruel and indifferent, when His thundering voice exclaimed, "Didn't I give you a child to hold and love? And didn't he reach up for you and call your name? And didn't he fill you with joy and excitement and renew your own ragged sense of wonder?"

"Yes, but why did you allow this to happen?" I demanded.

"Because wisdom and strength and love are also born of suffering. Is that so hard to understand? Must everything be perfect to satisfy you?"

Embarrassed by my greed and ignorance, I fell silent.

"Watch."

Suddenly, it was the Judgment Day, and all of the children with broken hearts and twisted and lifeless limbs were being swept up from their hospital beds and wheelchairs to join hands before us in a furious golden dance. One by one, they began to run and jump, soaring and whirling and rolling like acrobats and ballet dancers and gymnasts, while their parents formed a circle around them clapping their hands. And when they were finally exhausted, the children turned toward their parents, walking ever so slowly but erectly, with outstretched hands. "Did you like it?" I heard you ask.

When I opened my eyes, they were burning, and I saw we were over the river, hurtling through the morning fog toward Philadelphia. I do not think the person sitting next to me noticed that I was crying.

—JOURNAL ENTRY
AUGUST 19, 1991

The sky is still bloodied in the west, all ruse and incident, as we gather for our game. Meanwhile, the real action is taking place high above us, where night slips into position without protest, speckled and iridescent, like the color of a starling's tumescent belly.

Our noisy gaggle comprises an even dozen, four adults and eight children, some of whom are borrowed from other houses. As is customary, rules are sketchy and voices pitched. Gregory, I notice, has a politician's flair for washing over complicated questions with oratory. Cary, on the other hand, is an excellent listener, bobbing excitedly on his crutches, waiting for the signal to go.

"Okay, who's going to be the first ghost?" I ask.

"I am," Matt, an eighth grader, says. Then, like that, he is gone.

"Start counting," Greg calls.

Soon, we are flying into the night, raucous goblins all, in search of a solitary ghost muffled in the cooling shadows. The thought crosses my mind that in less than a dozen hours most of these children will be settling into another school year, nervous with new teachers and routines, even while the corpse of another summer is still warm.

When it is Cary's turn to be the ghost, I shoo the other children in the opposite direction, advising them to take five. Then I start into the heavy shadows that pin down our backyard.

"Whoooo." A tiny voice crackles at me from the direction of our storage shed in the corner.

"Now I wonder where that little ghost could be?" I whisper.

"Whooooo."

"Don't scare me like that, ghost."

Giggles now, and the familiar nervous clicking Cary's braces make when he bends his knees.

"I think I'm getting closer," I say as I push past the pine trees alongside of the shed.

"Boo, Daddy!" Cary shouts, suddenly hopping from beside the shed.

"Cary, I mean, ghostie, you scared me half to death."

Even in the dark I see Cary's face beaming. Luminous with pride, he casts off sparks, like tracers or shooting stars.

Every couple of steps on our way back, Cary stops to ask again, "Daddy, did I scare you?" And the way he asks, it is unclear who scared whom.

"You sure did," I assure him. "You gave me a great big scare."

"But you're not scared anymore?"

"Not anymore."

"Good."

"How about you?"

"I'm not scared."

"Good."

"Daddy?"

"Yeah, Cary?"

"I'm going to speed ahead back to the kids."

"Okay, I'll see you in a minute," I say, watching him hop ahead, disappearing around the corner of our house and under the whispering trees. "Watch out for ghosts," I call then. But he is gone already, out of earshot.

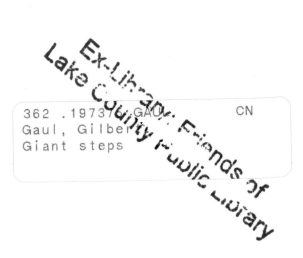
LAKE COUNTY PUBLIC LIBRARY
INDIANA

AD	FF	MU
AV	GR	NC
BO	HI	SC
CL	HO	SJ
DY	LS	FEB 2 3 '93 CN L

THIS BOOK IS RENEWABLE BY PHONE OR IN PERSON IF THERE IS NO RESERVE
WAITING OR FINE DUE.   LCP #0390